PREVENTION AND
CARE OF
ATHLETIC INJURIES
THIRD EDITION

James M. Booher, Ph.D., A.T.C., R.P.T.
Athletic Trainer and Professor
South Dakota State University
Brookings, South Dakota

eddie bowers publishing, inc.
2600 Jackson Street
Dubuque, Iowa 52001-3342

Exclusive marketing and distributor rights for
U.K., Eire, and Continental Europe held by:

   Gazelle Book Services Limited
   Falcon House
   Queen Square
   Lancaster LA1 1RN U.K.

eddie bowers publishing, inc.
2600 Jackson Street
Dubuque, Iowa 52001-3342 USA
eddiebowerspub@hotmail.com

ISBN 0-945483-40-6

CONTENTS

PREFACE

This manual is designed to cover the basic concepts of the management of athletic related injuries. It is intended for use in an introductory level course in athletic injuries. This manual is designed for coaches and teachers who will have the initial responsibility for the medical care of their teams. It is not intended for athletic training curriculums or to encompass all aspects of athletic training.

This manual is divided into six units. Unit 1 is concerned with the basic foundations of athletic injuries. Unit 2 discusses the various athletic injuries and a basic assessment process used to evaluate these injuries. Unit 3 discusses the common athletic injuries or conditions which may occur to the lower extremities, Unit 4 the axial region, and Unit 5 the upper extremities. Unit 6 discusses heat related conditions. With each body part covered, this manual will review the basic anatomy of the area, the more common athletic related injuries, the usual mechanisms causing these injuries, and common taping procedures used to provide support to these areas of the body. Taping procedures are illustrated in a step-by-step approach to make learning these procedures easier.

The majority of illustrations in this manual were created by the author. However, some of the illustrations are reprinted with permission from: Booher, JM and Thibodeau, GA; Athletic Injury Assessment, ed 2, 1989, CV Mosby.

BASIC FOUNDATIONS OF ATHLETIC INJURIES

The first unit of this manual discusses the basic foundations of athletic injuries. Included in this unit is a review of basic anatomy, a discussion of the body's response to trauma, and the standard procedures commonly used to manage athletic injuries.

ANATOMY REVIEW

The successful management of athletic injuries requires a fundamental understanding of human anatomy. The initial section of this manual deals with a review of the basic anatomy necessary for a student enrolled in an introductory prevention and care of athletic injuries course.

HUMAN SKELETON

The human skeleton is a joined framework of living organs called bones. The skeleton lies buried within the muscles and other soft tissues, thus providing a support structure for the body. The adult skeleton is composed of 206 separate bones. Rare variations in the total number of bones present in the body may occur as a result of certain anomalies such as extra ribs or from failure of certain bones to fuse in the course of development. The 206 bones are grouped into two subdivisions, namely the axial skeleton (80 bones) and the appendicular skeleton (126 bones). The axial skeleton includes six tiny middle ear bones and the 74 bones that form the upright axis of the body, including the skull, vertebral column, and thorax. The 126 bones of the appendicular skeleton form the appendages and girdles that attach them to the axial skeleton. Bones in each component of the skeleton can be reviewed in Figure 1-1 and are listed in Table 1-1.

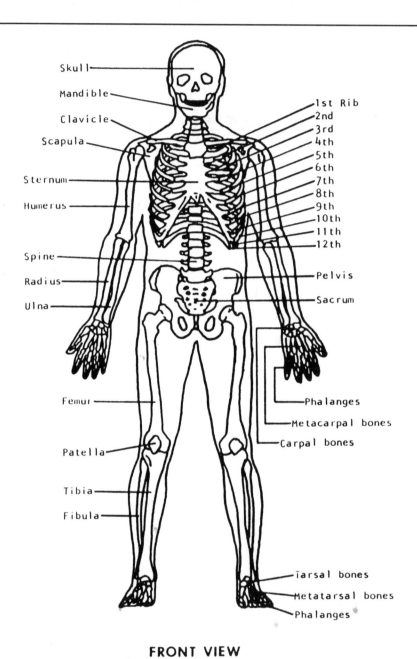

Skull
Mandible
Clavicle
Scapula
Sternum
Humerus
Spine
Radius
Ulna
Femur
Patella
Tibia
Fibula

1st Rib
2nd
3rd
4th
5th
6th
7th
8th
9th
10th
11th
12th
Pelvis
Sacrum
Phalanges
Metacarpal bones
Carpal bones
Tarsal bones
Metatarsal bones
Phalanges

FRONT VIEW

Fig.1-1a. Human skeleton.

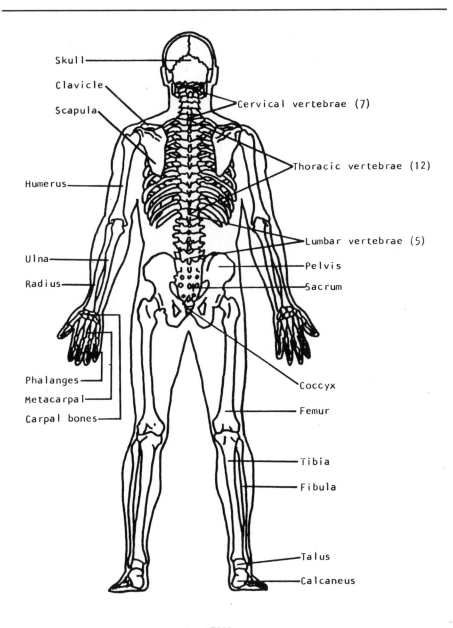

Skull

Clavicle

Scapula

Cervical vertebrae (7)

Thoracic vertebrae (12)

Humerus

Lumbar vertebrae (5)

Ulna

Pelvis

Radius

Sacrum

Phalanges

Metacarpal

Coccyx

Carpal bones

Femur

Tibia

Fibula

Talus

Calcaneus

BACK VIEW

Fig.1-1b. Human skeleton.

Bones in the Human Skeleton

Area	Number of Bones	Area	Number of Bones
AXIAL SKELETON		**APPENDICULAR SKELETON**	
Skull		Shoulder girdle	
Cranium	8	Clavicle	2
Face	14	Scapula	2
Hyoid	1	Upper extremities	
Ear ossicles	6	Humerus	2
Vertebral column		Ulna	2
Cervical vertebrae	7	Radius	2
Thoracic vertebrae	12	Carpals	16
Lumbar vertebrae	5	Metacarpales	10
Sacrum	1 (5 fused)	Phalanges	28
Coccyx	1 (3-5 fused)	Hip girdle	
Sternum	1	Innominate	2
Ribs	24	Lower extremities	
		Femur	2
		Tibia	2
		Fibula	2
		Patella	2
		Tarsals	14
		Metatarsals	10
		Phalanges	28
TOTAL BONES	80	**TOTAL BONES**	126

Table 1-1

JOINTS or ARTICULATIONS

A **joint** or **articulation** exists where two or more bones come together or meet. An understanding of articulations is important in understanding how joints function normally and in providing a basis for understanding the mechanics and nature of joint injuries. Athletic activities are characterized by complex, highly coordinated, and purposeful movements. Without an articulated skeleton, these movements would be impossible. Therefore, an overview of the classification, structure, and function of joints precedes the discussion of specific joint injuries.

Classification of Joints

Joints are classified into three major groups or types using either structural features or potential for movement as distinguishing criteria (Table 1-2). For our purposes, a system of joint classification using degree of movement is the more functional and appropriate method. The three joint classes are: synarthroses (immovable joints), amphiarthroses (slightly movable joints), and diarthroses (freely movable joints).

Joint Classification

Functional name	Structural name	Degree of movement permitted	Example
Synarthroses	Fibrous	Immovable	Sutures in skull
Amphiarthroses	Cartilaginous	Slightly movable	Pubic symphysis
Diarthroses	Synovial	Freely movable	Shoulder joint

Table 1-2

There are three basic types of synarthrotic or immovable joints. One is characterized by the presence of a dense fibrous membrane that binds the articular bone surfaces very closely and tightly to each other called a syndesmosis joint. Ligaments play an important role in restriction of movement in these joints. The articulation between the distal ends of the tibia and fibula is a good example of a **syndesmosis** joint.

The sutures of the skull are immovable joints formed by a series of jagged, interlocking processes of adjoining bone margins. The articulations between the roots of the teeth and sockets of the jaw bones are another example of a fibrous joint.

Amphiarthroses, or slightly movable joints, have a pad of fibrocartilage located between adjoining bony surfaces. The pubic symphysis or the joints between the ribs and the sternum are examples of an amphiarthrodial joints.

The diarthrotic or freely movable joints are often called synovial joints because they are characterized by the presence of a closed cavity or joint cavity lined with synovial membrane between the bones. These joints include by far the majority of the body's articulations. Synovial joints differ in strength or stability from one another depending upon the (1) skeletal or bony configuration, (2) ligamentous network, and (3) muscular arrangement. As each section of the body is described later in this manual, the relative strengths of major joints in the body will be discussed in more detail. Because they are the most mobile of the three types of joints, synovial joints are functionally the most important. They are also the most complex structure and are most vulnerable to athletic injuries. The structural features of synovial joints are illustrated in Figure 1-2.

Section Through a Synovial Joint

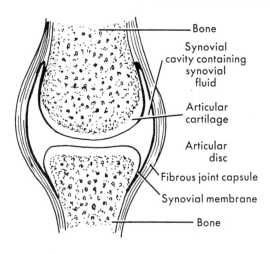

Bone

Synovial cavity containing synovial fluid

Articular cartilage

Articular disc

Fibrous joint capsule

Synovial membrane

Bone

Fig. 1-2

Fibrous joint capsule - a tough, dense but flexible sleevelike structure that helps join the articulating bones together. The capsule connects the periosteal membrane of one bone in the joint to that of the other and encloses a space that exists between the opposing bone surfaces. This space is called the **joint cavity**.

Synovial membrane - the deep or cellular inner layer of the joint capsule. This moist and slippery membrane lines the joint space between opposing bones and attaches to the margins of the articular cartilage. The function of the synovial membrane is to secrete **synovial fluid** which lubricates the joint and provides nourishment for the articular cartilage. This fluid resembles egg white in consistency and appearance.

Articular cartilage - a thin, gristlelike material that is firmly fixed to the ends of bones. The resiliency of the articular or **hyaline** cartilage cushions jars and blows that might otherwise erode or damage opposing bone surfaces in movable joints. The hyaline cartilage obtains its nutrients and oxygen from the synovial fluid in the joint space.

Articular discs - in addition to the thin layer of hyaline cartilage that covers the articulating surfaces in movable joints, pads of fibrocartilage may lie between the bones and divide the joint cavity. These pads are called **menisci**. They provide an additional "cushion" between the articulating ends of the bones and increase the stability of the joint. Torn or damaged fibrocartilage in a joint quite often does not heal properly and must be removed surgically. In most instances, only the damaged portion is removed, thus saving as much of the structure as possible.

Ligaments - strong cords of dense white fibrous tissue that grow between the bones, securing them together even more firmly than is possible with the joint capsule. Ligaments are invaluable in maintaining the anatomical integrity and structural alignment of a joint.

Types of Synovial Joints

Synovial joints are subdivided on the basis of (1) the kind of movement each joint is capable of performing and (2) the shape of the surfaces of the adjacent articulating bones. Table 1-3 lists the six types of synovial joints that can be grouped into three categories according to axial movement.

Classification of Synovial Joints

Axial Movement	Types	Examples
Uniaxial	Hinge	Elbow, knee, and ankle joints
	Pivot	Joint between first and second cervical vertebrae
Biaxial	Saddle	Joint between first metacarpal (thumb) and carpal bone
	Condyloid	Joint between radius and carpal bones
Multiaxial	Ball-and-Socket	Hip and shoulder joints
	Gliding	Joints between carpal and tarsal bones

Table 1-3

Uniaxial joints permit movement in only one plane and around a single axis. There are two types of uniaxial joints: hinge and pivot. Special mention should be made concerning hinge joints where only flexion and extension movements occur. Some examples in the body are the ankle, knee, elbow, and finger joints. Because they allow movement in only one plane and restriction in others, hinge joints are those most often involved in athletic injuries.

In biaxial joints, movement occurs in two planes and around two axes that are at right angles to each other. Flexion and extension are allowed around one axis and abduction and adduction around the second axis.

Multiaxial joints permit movement in all planes of the body. They include the ball-and-socket and gliding types of joints. Of all the joints in our body, the ball-and-socket joints permit the widest and freest range of movement. The gliding joints are numerous and almost always small. These joints allow the simplest type of movements, that is, slight displacement motion between the articular surfaces.

Review the movements and planes of the body, using the following list of definitions.

Position of the Body

Anatomical Position - standardized position in which the body is erect, facing forward and arms at the side with the palms of the hands turned forward.

Planes of the Body

Frontal plane - runs from side to side and divides the body into anterior (front) and posterior (back) portions.

Sagittal plane - runs from front to back and divides the body into right and left portions.

Transverse plane - crosswise section that divides the body into superior (upper) and inferior (lower) portions.

Movements of the Body

Flexion - decreasing the size of the angle between the anterior or posterior surfaces of articulated bones. An exception to this definition is the shoulder joint.

Extension - return from the flexed position.

Hyperextension - continuation of extension beyond the anatomical position.

Plantar flexion - movement of the sole of the foot downward.

Dorsiflexion - movement of the top of the foot upward.

Abduction - movement of a body part away from the midline of the body.

Adduction - movement of a body part toward the midline of the body.

Horizontal abduction - movement of the upper limb through the transverse plane at shoulder level away from the midline of the body.

Horizontal adduction - movement of the upper limb through the transverse plane at shoulder level toward the midline of the body.

Radial flexion - movement at the wrist of the thumb side of the hand toward the forearm.

Ulnar flexion - movement at the wrist of the little finger side of the hand toward the forearm.

Circumduction - composite movement, combining flexion, ab-duction, extension, and adduction, in which the body segment describes a cone.

Rotation - pivoting of a body part on its own central or longitu-dinal axis.

Pronation - turning the palms downward or backward.

Supination - turning the palms upward or forward.

Eversion - sole of the foot is turned outward.

Inversion - sole of the foot turned inward.

Elevation - upward movement of the shoulder complex.

Depression - return of movement from an elevated position.

Gliding - simplest type of movement involving slight relative displacement between adjoining bone surfaces.

SKELETAL MUSCLES

We have reviewed the basic architectural plan of the skeletal system and the joints or articulations that make the potential for move-ment possible. However, they cannot move themselves. They must be moved by the contraction of muscle tissue. Skeletal muscles comprise 40% - 50% of our body weight and attach to bones making movement possible.

There are over 600 skeletal muscles in the body and each can be thought of as a separate organ. However, muscles normally act in co-ordinated groups and not as single units. They tend to function in pairs, or in sets of three, four, or more in performing specific actions. Muscles vary significantly in size, shape, and fiber arrangement. They all have the same function, however, and behave in the same way; that is, they shorten. As muscles fibers shorten, their ends are pulled toward the center and contractile force or tension is developed which results in movement through a leverage system of the bones and joints.

Skeletal muscles normally attach to bones by a strong, tough fibrous tissue called **tendon.** Because tendons are stronger than the muscles they serve, injuries commonly occur within the muscle fibers, the musculotendinous junction or at the bony attachments. Certain tendons are enclosed in a tubular structure of fibrous connective tis-sue, called a **tendon sheath.** These sheaths have a lining of synovial membrane to enable the tendon to glide through the sheath almost fric-tionless.

Skeletal muscles are named on the basis of one or more distinctive features or characteristics such as, function, direction if its fibers, location, number of divisions, shape, size, or points of attachment. Refer to an anatomy book to review the names and locations of muscles. Some of the more important muscles will be reviewed in more detail in this manual with each body area.

PREVENTION OF ATHLETIC INJURIES

The best method of managing and caring for athletic injuries is to prevent them from occurring. Therefore, much of the coach's or athletic trainer's time should be devoted to preventing injuries. Numerous factors which are important in the prevention of athletic injuries are included in the following list.

Preparticipation examination
  Medical history
  Physical examination
  Fitness screening

Proper conditioning

Protective equipment
  Selection
  Fitting
  Maintenance

Safety supervision
  Facilities
  Equipment

Preventive techniques
  Taping
  Padding
  Bandaging
  Bracing

Monitoring environmental
  conditions

Observing athletes
  Recognize problems and minor
    injuries

Hygiene
  Rest
  Diet

Assessment techniques
  Recognizing injury
  Determining severity of injury
  Observation when returned to
    activity

Emergency care procedures
  Supplies
  Plan of action
  Immediate care

Rehabilitation strategies
  Prevent reinjury
  Strengthen previously injured
    area

THE BODY'S RESPONSE TO TRAUMA

To become competent and efficient in managing athletic injuries, you must possess a fundamental knowledge of how the body responds to various types of traumas and stresses associated with athletic activity. Athletic injuries normally result from some type of physical trauma, but can be caused by other circumstances such as infectious agents or exposure to hot or cold environments. The information in this section will enable you to better understand how the body responds to athletic related trauma.

When the body is subjected to injurious trauma or stress, it will usually respond in a systematic and predictable manner. The responses are essentially the same for all types of athletic injuries; that is, the process of inflammation and healing. Although these phenomena are not completely or clearly understood, the physiological and anatomical changes that characterize each step are reliable and predictable indicators about the initial injury and the subsequent course of the recovery process.

The body's response to a traumatic athletic injury is illustrated in Figure 1-3. This cycle outlines the sequence of events following an injury through the inflammatory and healing processes. Ideally, the end result is optimal recovery. Of course, depending on the severity of the injury and the management procedures used, this cycle can vary greatly in its length and conclude in less than optimal recovery and possibly reinjury or permanent loss of function.

The majority of athletic injuries are caused by some type of trauma, such as a direct blow, rotational stress, forced abnormal motion and overstretching or tearing forces. When these forces are greater than the tissues can withstand, varying degrees of damage result. Athletic trauma may involve the skin, muscles, tendons, ligaments, bones or nerves. A certain amount of hemorrhaging or bleeding will also be present if capillaries or other blood vessels are damaged. This bleeding may be external, if there is an open wound, or internal, if there is no break in the continuity of the skin. The body responds to hemorrhage by activating the clotting mechanism in an attempt to control the bleeding. In this type of injury there is also at least some direct cell damage as a result of the trauma. Cells that are damaged or torn lose their nutrition and, as a result, the ability to maintain the necessary cellular activities required for normal function. These dead tissue cells and the blood remaining outside the blood vessels as a result of hem-

Cycle of an Athletic Injury

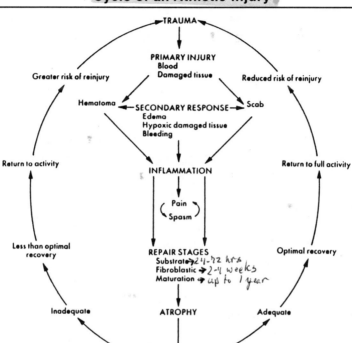

Fig. 1-3

orrhage will eventually develop into a mass called a **hematoma.** With open injuries, the blood and necrotic debris may form a thin blood clot, fill the apposed margins of the wounds, and subsequently form a scab on the surface.

The damaged tissue and blood resulting primarily from direct trauma are termed the initial insult or **primary injury.** Other than initiating procedures to bring bleeding under control as quickly as possible, you can have little if any effect on the extent of primary injury. Although it is considered the end of damage directly caused by initial trauma, swelling and tissue damage may not cease with the control of bleeding. Frequently, additional damage will occur that is secondary to the initial trauma or primary injury. This is called the secondary response or **secondary injury** and is discussed along with the inflammatory process. This phase of the athletic injury cycle can greatly be affected by the athletic trainer or coach.

ACUTE INFLAMMATORY PROCESS

The acute inflammatory process begins within minutes of the onset of injury. Inflammation is the basic response of vascularized tissues to an injurious agent, whether the source is physical, bacterial, thermal, or chemical. The inflammatory process is a nonspecific response designed to be the body's defense mechanism against trauma, regardless of cause. In athletics the most frequent cause of inflammation is physical trauma. The goal of the inflammatory proces is threefold: (1) to localize the extent of the injured area, (2) to rid both the body as a whole and the injury site of waste products resulting from the initial trauma and secondary responses, and (3) to enhance healing.

The initial phase of the acute inflammatory response is called the substrate stage and is characterized by localized vascular changes. After the injury there is an immediate transient constriction of local blood vessels, resulting in a decreased blood flow to the injured area. The initial vasoconstriction may last from 5 to 10 minutes, providing sufficient time for initial evaluation of the injury and transportation of the athlete off the field or court if necessary. This decreased flow of blood reduces the amount of oxygen and nutrients being delivered to the injury site and surrounding area and may cause cells uninjured by the initial trauma to be damaged by hypoxia. Cells that undergo secondary hypoxic death add to the debris from the initial injury, increasing the size of the hematoma. As a result of cells undergoing hypoxic death, the extent of the injury may be greater than that caused by the initial insult.

Transient vasoconstriction at the time of injury is followed by active vasodilation of local blood vessels, a rise in blood vessel hydrostatic pressure, and increased blood flow to the trauma site (Figure 1-4, B). Concurrent to this increased blood flow is congestion in the blood vessels and increased vascular permeability that allows the white blood cells, which have lined up along the vessel walls during vasoconstriction, to migrate toward the injury site (Figure 1-4, C). The increased vascular permeability, and any actual structural damage to blood vessels resulting from the injury, allow plasma and plasma proteins to leak out or escape from the blood vessels. This contributes to the collection of an excessive amount of blood fluids in the tissue spaces surrounding the blood vessels at the point of injury. This leakage of blood fluids accounts for much of the swelling (edema) associated with an injury and may continue for 24 to 48 hours, causing the injury site to be more extensive than that caused by the initial trauma.

Formation of Edema

A. Normal fluid, nutrient, and electrolyte exchange.

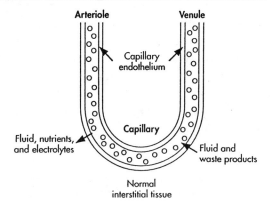

B. Initial edema formation as hydrostatic pressure and vessel permeability continues to increase.

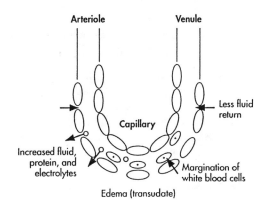

C. Edema formation continues as white blood cells, plasma proteins, and fluids escape the vessel.

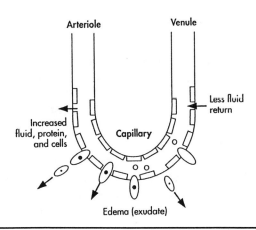

Fig. 1-4

The inflammatory process is an important defense mechanism that occurs for a specific purpose, namely to protect and heal an injured area. The signs and symptoms of inflammation, are (1) redness, (2) swelling, (3) heat, (4) pain, and (5) loss of function. These signs and symptoms serve to remind an athlete that he or she has been injured and are present to prevent the athlete from exceeding safe limits of activity and reinjuring the area. To effectively manage an injury, you must be able to recognize the signs and symptoms of inflammation and understand what they indicate.

Following is a brief explanation of these signs and symptoms and their causes:

Redness - caused by dilation of arterioles and increased flow of blood to the injured area.
Swelling - Caused by the accumulation of blood and damaged tissue cells in the primary injury area, as well as blood, hypoxic-damaged tissue debris, and edema resulting from the secondary reaction.
Heat - Caused by increased biochemical activity in the affected tissues and increased blood flow to the skin surface.
Pain - Caused by direct injury to nerve fibers as well as pressure of the hematoma or area of edema on nerve endings.
Loss of function - Caused by the resulting pain and swelling or the actual destruction of an anatomic structure, such as a fractured bone, ruptured ligament, or torn muscle.

The primary function of the inflammatory process in the days following an injury is to rid the area of waste products resulting from the primary and secondary responses in preparation for the healing process. As the blood vessels become more permeable and allow blood cells to migrate into the tissues, white blood cells infiltrate the injured area and concentrate at the injury site. In the early stages of the acute inflammatory response, these cells ingest and dispose of unwanted substances of the hematoma. After the debris is ingested, these white blood cells reenter the blood stream or lymphatic system and are carried away from the injury site. The successful completion of this activity usually marks the end of the acute inflammatory reaction. In most wounds not contaminated with bacteria or large amounts of foreign material, the acute inflammatory process subsides within several days, and the repair process continues to evolve.

Pain-Spasm Cycle

An additional response to trauma is the pain-spasm cycle. Generally, pain and muscle spasm of varying degrees accompany musculoskeletal injuries. Muscle spasm is a protective mechanism, designed to prevent further damage to an already injured area. The body attempts to splint the area surrounding the injury through the involuntary contraction of muscles or groups of muscles. The resulting contraction is called **muscle spasm**. As the muscle spasm develops, there is increased pressure on the nerve endings, resulting in more pain. The body responds to the increased pain with increased muscle spasms, resulting in more pain, and so on; hence the name pain-spasm cycle.

THE PROCESS OF WOUND HEALING

The process of wound healing begins with the acute inflammatory reaction and then accelerates when enough of the hematoma has been removed to permit the growth of new tissue. The formation of new tissue is required to replace tissues that were damaged by the injury. Most tissues involved in athletic injuries do not have the ability to regenerate their respective specialized cells, and instead undergo a relatively nonspecific repair process, that of **scar formation**. Our epidermis and bones, however, do have the ability to regenerate,or heal, with the same type of tissue that was damaged. Unfortunately, most soft tissues in the body heal with the formation of scar tissue, which is less than an ideal replacement. Scar formation is virtually identical in all tissues of the body. However, the final appearance of a scar and its effect on function will vary, depending on the tissue involved and the treatment given. Treatment and rehabilitation procedures differ somewhat between various types of tissues injured.

The removal of most of the necrotic debris from the injury site is followed by development of a dense network of capillaries early in the healing process. Along with the formation of this capillary network, **fibroblasts**, which are connective tissue cells that form the fibrous connective tissues in the body, proliferate in the damaged area. This phase of wound healing of scar formation is known as **fibroplasia**. These fibroblasts manufacture collagen, which is the main supportive protein in skin, tendon, bone, cartilage, and connective tissue. Significant amounts of collagen are laid down by the fourth or fifth day after an injury, so that a loose mesh of fibrous connective tissue occupies the injured area. This connective tissue is vascular and fragile. The phenomenon of fibroblast proliferation and collagen accumulation after injury usually continues for 2 to 4 weeks. During this time the vascularity of the new fibrous connective tissue continues to decrease, and the tensile strength increases. As a sufficient quantity of collagen is produced, the number of fibroblasts in the wound diminishes. The disappearance of these fibroblasts marks the end of the fibroplastic phase and the beginning of the **maturation phase**.

During the maturation phase of wound healing, pronounced changes occur in the newly formed fibrous connective tissue. The scar that is formed during fibroplasia is an enlarged and dense but unorganized structure of collagen. The fibers of collagen are initially randomly arranged but in time will line up along lines of stress. The union between the damaged tissues is still moderately fragile. During the next several months, the strength of the scar continues to increase and the collagen fibers change to a more organized pattern. As the scar tissue matures, it shrinks and becomes avascular and acellular. This maturation process may continue for a year or longer.

It is important to understand the basic fundamentals of wound repair and scar formation to gain optimum treatment results and achieve full recovery with injured athletes. Remember, your responsibility may be to localize the inflammatory response, promote the healing process, and ensure that athletes are not imposing undue stresses on healing tissue that is not mature or ready for strenuous activity.

Open wounds, those involving a break in the continuity of the skin, should be thoroughly cleansed to remove any foreign material, obvious necrotic tissue, or bacterial contaminants. Wound healing that occurs in the absence of infection is called **healing by first intention**. If infection with pus formation does occur, there will be little if any healing until the infection is overcome. This is called **healing by second intention**. Wound edges must be restored as closely as possible to normal anatomic relationships to minimize both the amount of fibroplasia required for healing to occur and the width of the resulting scar. Although this is primarily a physician's responsibility, you maybe called on to protect the injured area when the athlete returns to activity and to inspect the wound periodically to ensure that it does not reopen or become infected.

Athletic injuries involving structures deep to the skin must be treated to heal in such a way that function of the involved anatomic part will be restored to an optimum level. In many instances when a structure is ruptured or torn, it is desirable to repair it surgically. The goal of surgical repair is to bring the ruptured ends together so that a shorter distance has to be spanned by scar tissue. The injured area must be protected from abnormal stresses, which can interfere with the healing process and weaken, stretch, or tear the developing scar tissue and result in loss of function or instability. This protection or immobilization may be in the form of a cast, brace, splint, tape, or rest.

Rehabilitation procedures will differ, depending on the type of tissues injured. Injuries involving the contractile unit (muscles and tendons) are treated and managed differently that those involving noncontractile tissues such as ligaments. If muscles and tendons are allowed to heal without active early motion, it may be very difficult to restore full range of motion. Range of motion exercises should be started as early as possible once swelling and tenderness have subsided to the point that exercises are not unduly painful. However, starting too early may impede the healing process, cause additional hemorrhage and swelling, and result in a bigger scar and possibly a limitation in function. Allowing the musculotendinous unit to heal in a shortened state will result in a loss of motion, requiring constant stretching and making the athlete more vulnerable to repeated strains. These contractile tissues may require a certain amount of support and protection when activity is resumed. Occasionally injuries to the contractile unit will result in the formations of fibrous **adhesions** that bind the tendon or muscle to surrounding tissues and interfere with normal movement.

Ligament injuries require a long period of time (possibly 6 months) to heal to the point of regaining near normal tensile strength. If ligaments are subjected to abnormal stresses early in the healing process, the developing scar tissue may elongate, resulting in some degree of permanent instability of the involved joint. External means of protection or immobilization, such as a cast, brace, or taping, are used until the healing ligament is moderately strong and the surrounding muscles can be rehabilitated to assist in the support of the joint. In many cases the injured joint will require continued support and protection when athletic activity is resumed.

Another result of the injury cycle that you must be aware of is **atrophy**. Atrophy is the wasting away or deterioration of a tissue, organ, or part. During the healing process, if the injured area has been immobilized or otherwise inactive, atrophy will occur. In most cases the degree of atrophy is directly proportional to the amount and time of immobilization. Occasionally, changes in vascularity and innervation of a body area will also result in atrophy. Regardless of cause, an area of the body that has atrophied is more susceptible to reinjury, thus instigating repetition of the injury cycle. Therefore the injured athlete should not be returned to full athletic activity until the area has been rehabilitated to an optimal level.

PSYCHOLOGICAL RESPONSES TO TRAUMA

Another phenomenon you must consider with any athletic injury is the psychologic responses of the athlete to physical trauma and pain. Athletes perceive physical trauma in different ways. Perceived changes in body habitus, gait, appearance, and functional ability all contribute to the psychologic reality of injury. Some may perceive an athletic injury as a disaster, whereas others may find it a welcome relief from poor performance, a losing season, or lack of playing time. Athletes can undergo a variety of psychologic reactions to an injury, such as anger, disbelief, denial, alienation, depression, isolation, resignation, or acceptance. In fact, an athlete may go through all of these reactions during a single injury situation. Some of these reactions can develop into a self-defeating attitude and become blocking forces to effective recovery and rehabilitation. Athletes may lack motivation to recover and wonder if they ever will completely recover and compete again. Although it is not the purpose of this manual to discuss complex psychologic mechanisms of human behavior, you must be aware that these factors can greatly affect the physiological responses to trauma. Recovery depends on the proper psychological attitude as well as on the physiological processes involved. It is recommended you combine sound physiological treatment techniques with a positive, encouraging attitude in an attempt to effectively treat the mind as well as the body.

CHRONIC INFLAMMATION

Chronic is defined as long lasting. Although there is no sharp delineation of time between acute and chronic, **acute** generally refers to a matter of hours or days, whereas chronic refers to weeks, months, or years. **Chronic inflammation** may result from overuse, improper technique, continued stress, or repeated injury to a structure or area of the body. For whatever reason, the inflammatory response continues to repeat itself and can be detrimental to an athlete's performance. Such conditions as tennis elbow, jumper's knee, stress fractures, and shin splints are typical examples of chronic inflammatory conditions. They can progress to a point at which they disable an athlete. Although these seem to be different conditions, chronic inflammatory responses are basically alike and require similar treatment; rest, local heat, protection against reinjury, modification of activity, and perhaps anti-inflammatory medications prescribed by a physician. In chronic overuse conditions, identification of possible causes and preventive measures is very important.

The purpose of any training program is to build up the body's structures gradually so they are able to withstand progressively heavier workloads, thus increasing their strength, endurance, and ability to avoid injury. Once a chronic inflammatory condition occurs, it is up to you, the coach and/or a physician to attempt to identify and eliminate the possible causes. These problems can be magnified by the fact that in many cases relief will require a sharp reversal of activity. A period of complete rest may be required, which must then be followed by a gradual increase in workload. This can become very frustrating and burdensome to the athlete and/or coach, especially if the injury occurs during the athletic season. The athlete's impatience to resume activity too soon or at too great an intensity level often results in recurrence of the condition and an even more frustrating period of disability.

SHOCK

Another of the body's responses to trauma is **shock**. Shock is a state of collapse or depression of the cardiovascular system. It does not occur very often in athletics; however, any significant athletic injury can result in shock. The possibilities of shock developing are much greater with severe bleeding (external or internal), spinal injuries, major fractures, or significant intrathoracic or intra-abdominal injuries. There are three main causes of shock: (1) the heart is damaged so that it fails to pump properly, (2) blood is lost so that there is an insufficient volume of fluid in the circulatory system, and (3) blood vessels dilate so that blood "pools" in the larger vessels, resulting in a diminished amount of fluid available to provide efficient circulation. One of these last two causes are most often responsible for shock when it occurs because of athletic injuries.

The result of shock is the same no matter what the cause; that is, a diminished amount of fluid available in the circulatory system. This results in an insufficient perfusion of blood providing oxygen and nutrients through the tissues and organs of the body. All bodily processes are affected. Body systems are depressed, and vital functions slow down. Shock is always serious; if this condition is not treated properly and promptly, death can result.

Shock develops in distinct stages. It can progress quite rapidly or develop over a period of hours. It is important to recognize the following signs and to be prepared to properly care for an injured athlete.

Stages of Shock

1. Rapid, weak pulse
2. Cool, clammy skin
3. Rapid, shallow breathing
4. Profuse sweating
5. Pale skin, and later, cyanotic mucous membranes
6. Nausea, possibly vomiting
7. Dull, lackluster eyes; pupils may dilate
8. Steadily falling blood pressure
9. Unconsciousness

As soon as you recognize any of these signs, the athlete should be treated for shock. Shock is a serious condition, but if recognized quickly and treated effectively, it can be reversed. The general treatment for shock is as follows:

Treatment of Shock

1. Establish and maintain a clear airway.
2. Control obvious bleeding.
3. Keep the athlete lying down, and elevate the lower extremities if the injury will not be aggravated. If there is a head, spinal, or abdominal injury or breathing difficulties, keep the athlete flat or in a comfortable position.
4. Maintain body temperature as near normal as possible. In cold temperatures, keep the athlete warm and reduce the loss of body heat.
5. Do not give anything to eat or drink.
6. Transport the athlete to medical facilities or summon medical assistance.

STANDARD PROCEDURES
OF INITIAL TREATMENT

The standard procedures for the immediate care of athletic injuries are based on how the body responds to trauma and the acute inflammatory process. These initial treatment procedures are designed to control the swelling and minimize the magnitude of the hematoma, which allows the process of healing to begin earlier and proceed at a more rapid rate. The standard procedure for the initial care of an athletic injury are universally accepted and can be remembered by the acronym ICERS. These letters stand for the steps of **Ice, Compression, Elevation, Rest**, and **Support** (Figure 1-5). Each of these steps is important and should not be overlooked when caring for an acute athletic injury.

Standard Procedure of Initial Care for an Athletic Injury:
Ice, Compression, Elevation, Rest, and Support

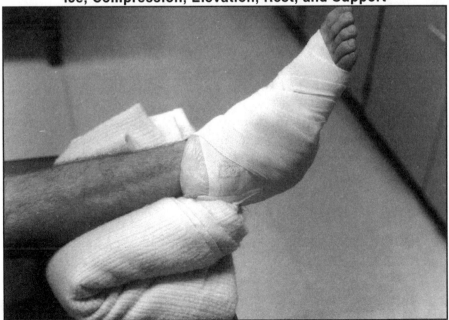

Fig. 1-5

ICE

The first step is to put some form of cold application on the injured area, whether it is an ice pack or cold immersion. Cold applied promptly after an injury can slow down or minimize some of the acute inflammatory reactions previously discussed. In addition, cold diminishes local blood flow and helps constrict capillaries in the area of injury. The local application of cold also decreases clotting time because it increases the viscosity of the fluids and decreases the rate of flow in the injured area. This quicker clotting reduces hemorrhaging in the area of injury. Another important effect of cold is to lower tissue temperature, thus decreasing the metabolic demands and slowing the chemical actions in cells surrounding the injured area. This reduces the build up of waste products in the area and allows more tissue cells to survive the period of temporary hypoxia. Cold applications are also beneficial in reducing the amount of muscle spasms that usually accompany athletic injuries. Therefore there is less discomfort associated with the pain-spasm cycle.

COMPRESSION

The purpose of compression on an acute injury is to help control or reduce the amount of edema and provide mild support. Compression about an injured area is normally accomplished by the use of an elastic wrap or appropriate taping. Compression acts as a physical deterrent to swelling by preventing fluids from accumulating in the injured area. Compression also increases the tissue pressure outside the blood vessels, thus helping to prevent edema caused by plasma seepage or extravasation. Normally, compression will also make an injured area feel more comfortable. Although an elastic wrap offers only mild support, the pressure does appear to provide some relief of pain. The fundamentals of compression bandaging are discussed and illustrated in Figures 1-11 through 1-17.

ELEVATION

Elevation of an injured area limits fluid pooling and encourages venous return. Elevating an injured area also decreases the hydrostatic pressure within the blood vessels, which helps decrease the amount of edema by decreasing the volume of fluid filtered out of the blood vessels and into the tissue spaces. Controlling the edema associated with an injured area decreases tissue damage and results in a smaller area to be repaired.

REST

Resting an injured area is necessary to allow the body time to get the effects of the trauma under control and to avoid additional stress and damage to injured tissue. The period of rest, required will vary, depending on the coach's, athletic trainer's, and physician's philosophy and on the severity of the injury. The length of rest may range from a 10-minute break in a practice to many months of postoperative recovery. Athletes who continue to participate with an acutely injured area may increase hemorrhage and the amount of initial tissue damage as well as the amount and severity of secondary injury response, such as edema formation and the accumulation of tissue debris from hypoxic damage. All of this can result in a larger hematoma, slower healing, and a longer recovery period.

SUPPORT

Another important aspect of the initial treatment is that of support and protection. Often an injury requires stabilization or immobilization to prevent further injury. The use of various materials, such as braces, splints, casts, tape, pads, or crutches all can be used to protect and support injured areas (Figure 1-6). Varying degrees of support or protection often have to be provided throughout the healing phase and perhaps longer. Remember, you are attempting to provide for optimum conditions for recovery during the healing phase.

The purpose of the initial treatment procedures of ice, compression, elevation, rest, and support is to minimize the effects of an injury at its onset and to create an optimal environment for healing, thereby reducing the loss of function and length of the recovery period. Normally these procedures are used for at least 2 to 3 days after a significant injury. Although you can do little to speed up the actual healing process, you can have a tremendous effect on the total recovery time and on the quality of the repair.

Injured Ankle Supported by Adhesive Tape

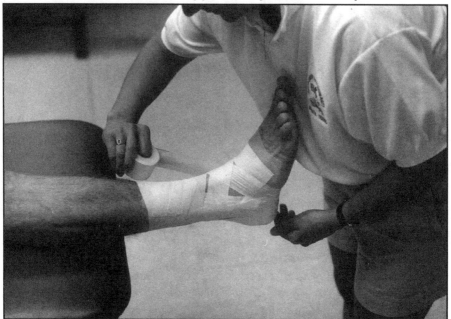

Fig. 1-6

FOLLOW-UP TREATMENT PROCEDURES

Treatment procedures used after the immediate postinjury period are designed to rehabilitate the athlete toward full functional use of the injured area and return him or her to an optimal level of performance in a minimal period of time. Both heat and cold modalities are used after the initial treatment period; however, heat should not be used until you are relatively sure no further bleeding or swelling will occur. Heat is used primarily to increase the circulation to an area. Cold is used primarily to relieve pain, thereby allowing early and more extensive range of motion. Both of these modalities should always be used in conjunction with some type of exercise. **Exercise** is the primary modality used to rehabilitate an injured area and is the most effective method of increasing blood flow to an area. The increased blood flow helps resolve the hematoma and deliver oxygen and nutrients required in rebuilding injured tissues. The specific use of heat and cold modalities is discussed in the next section.

If you have the responsibility for the health care of an athletic team, you must be familiar with rehabilitation procedures and assume a leadership role in convincing an injured athlete that the key to a good rehabilitation program is continued progressive exercise, not just an extension of passive treatment activity for a longer period of time. The type of exercises used to restore normal function depend on the nature and severity of the injury as well as the philosophy of the individual supervising the rehab. Today's rehab is sports specific and combines strength, flexibility, balance, and coordination. Exercises should be performed essentially pain free and progress as fast as possible from active range of motion to full participation. This may be completed in days or may take 3 to 4 weeks or longer. Pain is the primary governing force for all treatment procedures. As long as the exercise is pain free, the athlete should be encouraged to increase the level of activity. If the exercise is painful or if **residual swelling** and **pain** are present following treatment, the activity is too strenuous and should be modified.

THERAPEUTIC MODALITIES

Cold and heat treatment procedures are commonly used in treating athletic injuries. The physiological basis for these modalities was briefly discussed previously. This section is concerned with the specific methods of applying the more commonly used cold and heat modalities.

COLD THERAPY (CRYOTHERAPY)

Cold treatments are used for at least the first 48-72 hours following an athletic injury or as long as there is any danger of additional bleeding or swelling. Remember, cold is used initially to control swelling and relieve pain. However, there is some disagreement as to whether cold or heat is more beneficial in treating an injury after this initial period. Cold as a follow-up treatment procedure is used primarily for its pain relieving (**anesthetic**) effects. Cold is a more effective pain reliever than heat. When pain and muscle spasms are decreased, an athlete can exercise earlier and more effectively. Remember, the earlier a rehabilitative exercise program is started, the less chance there is for atrophy and the formation of adhesions. As mentioned previously, exercise is also a very effective method of increasing blood flow to an area. The increased blood flow to an injured site assists in ridding the body of the hematoma and delivers oxygen and nutrients to be used in the rebuilding process. The combination of cold and exercise is called **cryokinetics**. Studies have shown that cryokinetics result in a significant increase in blood flow when compared to heat alone. However, if exercises are too strenuous or begin too soon, enough pain will be experienced by the athlete to warrant stopping or modifying the exercises. Many times stretching techniques are included with or just following the application of cold.

Anyone using cold modalities must also remember that these treatments are usually not comfortable. There are four sensations an athlete will go through to obtain the maximum benefits from the cold treatment. Initially, the athlete will experience a sensation of (1) cold, which becomes increasingly uncomfortable or a (2) burning sensation, followed by an (3) aching feeling and then (4) anesthesia or numbness. Athletes may have to be reminded of these four sensations and that he or she must go through the first three steps before the area becomes numb.

Methods of Cold Application

There are many methods of applying cold to an injured area. Following is a brief description of the more commonly used methods.

Ice Pack - one of the easiest and most frequent methods of applying cold. A commercially prepared ice cap or plastic bag is filled with ice and placed upon the injured area as shown previously in Figure 1-5. Time of treatment is 15-20 minutes.

Cold Water Immersion - another commonly used method employing a tub, bucket, or whirlpool filled with cold water, with a temperature of less than 60°F (Figure 1-7). This is an effective treatment procedure for body areas such as the knee, ankle, elbow, or hand. Time of treatment is 15-20 minutes.

Ice Massage - method of treatment employs the use of a styrofoam or paper cup filled with water and frozen. The cup is torn away from the ice cube as it is used (Figure 1-8). The injured area is massaged with the ice until the athlete reports local numbness or anesthesia and the area is a pink color. This treatment usually takes approximately ten minutes and varies with the area and type of tissue

Cold Water Immersion

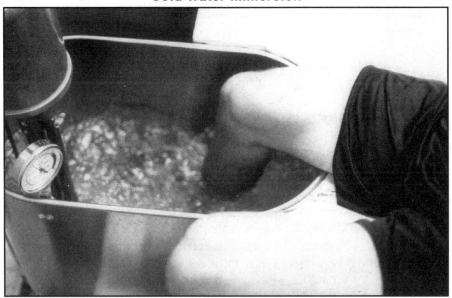

Fig. 1-7

Ice Massage

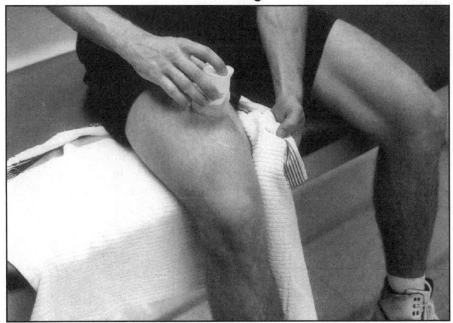

Fig. 1-8

being treated. The massaging action should be slow and gentle. An advantage of this technique is that athletes can usually administer treatment to themselves. A disadvantage is that it may be messy as the ice melts.

Cold Sprays - quite popular 10-20 years ago. The cooling effect does not last long enough and there is a danger of frostbite if too much is sprayed on.

Chemical Cold Packs - convenient to use, but are relatively expensive. They are not as cold or as long lasting as ice packs.

HEAT THERAPY (THERMOTHERAPY)

Heat has traditionally been used in treating athletic injuries following the initial 48 to 72 hours. The main effect of heat when applied to an area is an increase in local circulation. Remember, heat will increase swelling and should not be used until swelling has been controlled.

Methods of Heat Application

Following are methods of heat applications commonly used in the training room. All heat modalities should be applied so the athlete experiences a comfortably warm sensation. Time of treatment for heat modalities is 20-30 minutes.

Warm Water Immersion - warm water in a tub, bucket, or whirlpool. The temperatures should range between 100-108°F and are determined by the amount of body area in the water. The greater the body area in the water, the lower the temperature.

Heat Lamp - a 250 watt luminous heat bulb is most commonly used. The lamp is directed perpendicular to the injured area and is applied to bare, dry skin. The intensity of the heat is controlled by moving the lamp closer or farther away from the area. The normal distance is 18-20 inches.

Moist Heat Packs (hydrocollator) - a commercially prepared pack that is heated in water 140-160°F. The pack is then placed between layers of toweling (usually 6-8) and placed on the injured area (Figure 1-9). Intensity of the heat is controlled by the number of layers.

Applying a Moist Heat Pack

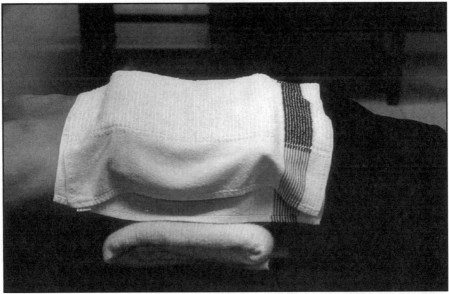

Fig. 1-9

These three methods are those most often used to apply heat to an injured area. All are fairly superficial. Occasionally electric heating pads, hot water bottles, or warm toweling are used.

Sometimes a deeper heat is indicated or prescribed for treatment, such as ultrasound or diathermy. These deeper penetrating modalities require additional training and a physician's prescription to use.

OTHER MODALITIES

Contrast Baths - alternating between warm and cold water. This produces a relaxation and contraction of the superficial blood vessels resulting in a mild shock to our circulatory system. Normally a treatment will last between 20-30 minutes and consist of alternating between warm and cold water at the rate of four minutes to one (Figure 1-10). Most effective on the hands or feet.

Contrast Bath Applied to an Ankle

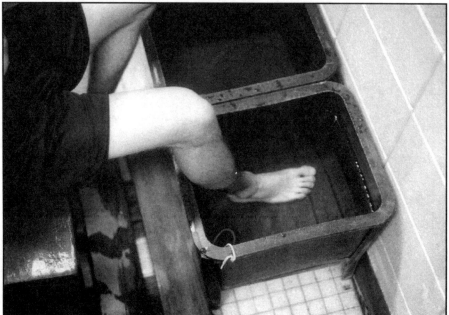

Fig. 1-10

Skin Counterirritants - are not as popular or used as much today as in the past. These include various liniments and analgesic balms which are very superficial and irritate or stimulate the skin. They give the feeling of warmth and may relieve mild pain by producing a stimulus to the skin of such intensity that the athlete is no longer aware of the feeling of pain. Skin counterirritants in no way replace a warm-up or heat treatment.

SUMMARY

The body's response to trauma is generally well established and programmed. When some type of trauma occurs, there is a certain amount of damaged tissue and blood that accumulates as the result of the primary injury. In addition to hematoma formation, there is frequently a secondary response that causes the injury site to become even more extensive. The secondary response includes edema and hypoxia and may continue for 24 to 48 hours. The body responds to this trauma with an inflammatory reaction designed to localize the extent of the injured area, rid the body of waste products, and enhance healing. The process of inflammation and healing form a continuum that can be subdivided into three phases; substrate (vascular changes and phagocytosis), fibroplastic (laying down of collagen fibers), and maturation (scar development). However, portions of these phases can occur simultaneously. For example, fibroplasia begins during the substrate phase, and scar maturation begins while collagen production continues. Possessing a fundamental knowledge of what happens to the body as a result of trauma provides you with a more rational basis for the management of various athletic injuries.

It is important to positively affect and influence the healing process to gain optimal treatment results with the injured athlete. This is initially accomplished through reducing the effects of the initial injury or trauma. Bleeding and swelling must be controlled as quickly as possible to minimize the magnitude of the hematoma. Limiting the hematoma allows the healing process to commence earlier, reducing the length of inactivity caused by the injury. Follow-up treatment procedures using exercise in conjunction with various methods of heat or cold applications are designed to optimally rehabilitate the injured athlete in a minimal period of time.

FUNDAMENTALS OF COMPRESSION BANDAGES

Compression (elastic) bandages are readily applicable in athletic training. They are often used to apply pressure to an injured body area which in turn increases the pressure outside the blood vessels to help control edema. They are also used to provide mild support for muscular types of injuries and to hold dressings, packs, or protective pads in place. Around movable joints, figure eight or spica techniques are used to maintain the wrap in proper position. The spica has a larger loop on one end than does the figure eight. The following diagrams illustrate how to apply elastic bandages to various areas of the body.

The foot and ankle wrap is used primarily to provide compression to the area following an injury. Using a 4" wrap, begin with an anchor around the foot at the toes (Figure 1-11, A). The wrap is then brought around the heel and back to the starting point (B). Repeat this figure eight procedure several times with each revolution progressing backward on the foot and upward on the leg. Each figure eight should overlap the preceding one by about 1/2 the width of the wrap (C). Finish by spiraling around the leg and lock with tape.

Foot and Ankle Figure Eight Wrap

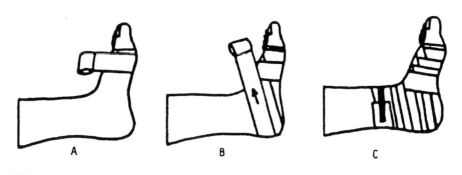

A   B   C

Fig. 1-11

The knee wrap is also used primarily to provide compression following an injury. Using a 6" wrap, anchor by one turn around the leg at approximately mid calf (Figure 1-12, A). The wrap is then brought across the inside of the knee joint and encircles the thigh approximately mid thigh (B). After one revolution around the thigh, the wrap is brought down across the knee joint again (C). The remaining wrap can now be spiraled up the leg overlapping 1/2 the preceding piece and locked with tape (D).

Knee Figure Eight Wrap

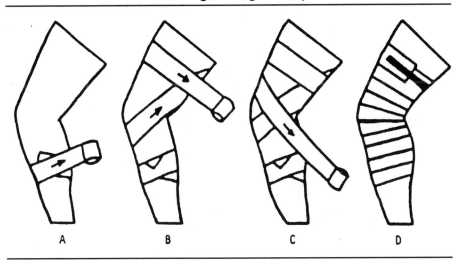

A   B   C   D

Fig. 1-12

Elastic wraps on the thigh are used for compression, mild support, or to hold a pack or protective pad in place. A 6" wrap should be used in a spiraling manner (Figure 1-13). Note in (A) that the wrap should begin in such a fashion that the beginning corner forms a flap that can be folded down and locked into the wrap. This is to prevent the wrap from coming loose at the bottom.

Thigh Wrap

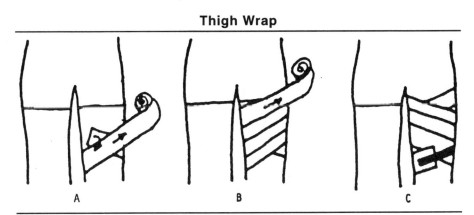

A   B   C

Fig. 1-13

Elastic wraps at the hip are most often used to provide mild support to injured muscles. A 6" wrap should be used. This is a body area where it is often benificial to use a double length 6" wrap. To support hip flexors or adductors (groin muscles), a **flexed hip spica** should be used. Instruct the athlete to place his or her foot on a bench or stool so the injured hip is flexed approximately 90° (Figure 1-14, A). Start with an anchor that encircles the upper thigh and pulls upward into the groin (B). The wrap is then taken around the waist and back around the upper thigh (C). At least two complete spicas should be made and the wrap secured around the thigh with tape (D).

Flexed Hip Spica Wrap

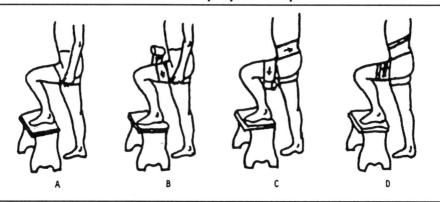

A   B   C   D

Fig. 1-14

To support high hamstring muscle strains, the hip spica is done with the athlete in a standing position. The wrap encircles the upper thigh so that the pull is toward the back or hamstring area (Figure 1-15, A). The wrap is then taken around the waist and back around the upper thigh (B). Again, at least two spicas should be made and the wrap secured around the thigh with tape (C).

Posterior Hip Spica Wrap

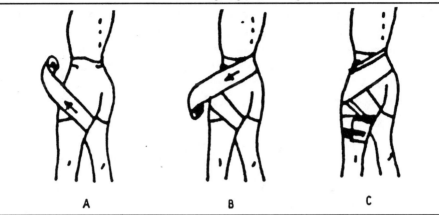

A   B   C

Fig. 1-15

The shoulder spica is used primarily for mild support. Using a 6" wrap, begin with an anchor around the upper arm (Figure 1-16, A). The wrap is then placed over the point of the shoulder, around the athlete's trunk, under the unaffected arm and back up over the injured shoulder (B). Two spicas should be made and the wrap secured with tape around the upper arm (C). The shoulder spica is often done with a double length wrap.

Shoulder Spica Wrap

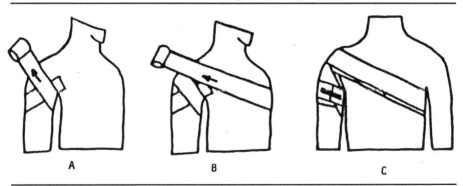

A   B   C

Fig. 1-16

The elbow figure eight is used primarily for providing compression following an injury. Using a 4" wrap, anchor the bandage around the forearm (Figure 1-17). Then bring the wrap across the front of the elbow joint and encircle the upper arm (A). After going around the arm at least once, continue the wrap back down across the elbow joint again (B). With the remaining wrap, spiral up the arm overlapping 1/2 the preceding strip and lock with tape (C).

Elbow Figure Eight Wrap

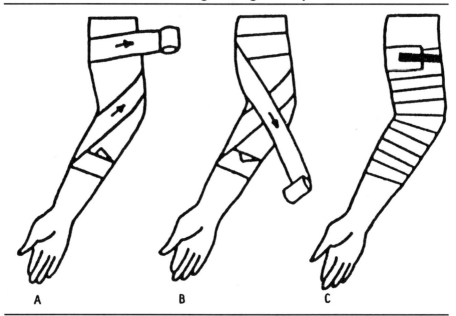

A   B   C

Fig. 1-17

FUNDAMENTALS OF ATHLETIC TAPING

The use of adhesive tape is a common occurrence around athletic teams. The primary uses can be summarized in the following list:

1. Stabilization of compression bandages protective padding or devices.
2. Securing dressings in place.
3. Protection against possible injury.
4. Support or protection of an injured or weakened area.

Two types of tape are normally used in athletic training, **linen** and **elastic**. Linen is non-elastic and most commonly used. It comes in various widths and is usually packaged in a case or speed pack, with each roll being 15 yards in length. The 1 1/2" or 2" widths are most commonly used in athletic training. Linen tape also comes in various grades according to the number of threads per square inch. The most commonly used tape is either 48 x 64 or 48 x 72 fibers per square inch.

Elastic tape also comes in rolls that are various widths and usually 5 yards in length. Some elastic tapes can be torn by hand are employed in a variety of uses. Other types of elastic tape must be cut with scissors and are usually more expensive. This type of tape is used primarily for support at highly movable joints such as the knee or elbow.

Listed below are the basic fundamentals of applying adhesive tape. Once these fundamentals are learned, you can improvise the application of tape to any area of the body. Common methods of applying tape are described and illustrated throughout the remainder of this manual.

1. The area to be taped should be clean and dry. Small traces of oil, powder, dust, moisture, or liniment interfere with the adhesion of adhesive tape.
2. The part of the body to be taped should be shaved. Maximum support is provided when tape is applied directly to the skin. However, daily taping can lead to skin irritation or athletes may disapprove of a body area being shaved. To overcome these types of problems, some type of underwrap material is often applied. In addition, it is often desirable to place protective pads over areas of high stress or sensi-

tive areas to prevent tape cuts or blisters. Examples of high stress areas are anterior to the ankle joint and the achilles tendon area. Sensitive areas include the back of the knee or front of the elbow.

3. A small amount of an adherent, which provides a tacky surface on which to tape, can also be applied. Tape adheres more firmly to this tacky surface.

4. The part of the body to be taped should be in a functional position. The body area should be placed in a position in which it is to be stabilized. Remember, to provide support using adhesive tape, you must take away some motion of the involved joint. Visualize what you want the tape to do or which direction you want to support. Each strip of tape should be laid with a particular purpose in mind. Your taping procedure must provide sufficient support and at the same time allow sufficient movement at the joint to permit the athlete to continue activity.

5. Use a tape size that fits the contour or area to be covered. The more acute the angles present and smaller the body part, the narrower the tape width needed to fit the area.

6. The tape should start with an anchor and finish with lock strips. The principle of taping is to "bridge" the injured area by starting and ending on an uninjured area.

7. The tape should fit the natural contour of the part being taped. Failure to fit the natural contours creates wrinkles and gaps that can result in skin irritations.

8. The tape should be smoothed and molded as it is laid on the skin in order to avoid wrinkles, because many times wrinkles may cause small blisters or abrasions under the tape. **Neatness** is the trademark of a good taper.

9. Tape should be applied snugly, but not so tightly as to constrict. Many times tape should be applied at the tension it comes off the roll.

10. Avoid continuous taping around a body part because this may cause constriction and makes it more difficult to follow the natural contours of the area.

11. Each strip should overlap at least one-half the width of the preceding piece so that open areas do not form during activity which may cause skin irritations.

12. Keep the roll of tape in your hand and tear it with your fingers (Figure 1-18). Time is wasted by putting the tape down after each strip is torn or by cutting tape with scissors. However, many elastic tapes do require the use of scissors.
13. Remove tape carefully by pulling it parallel to the skin, rather than outward or away from it to avoid skin irritations.
14. The skin should be cleaned and checked for irritation following the removal of tape. Any skin irritation or rash should be treated immediately.

Tearing Tape

Learning to tear tape effectively is essential for speed and efficiency of taping. The secret of tearing tape is to break the first thread. Strength is not necessary to tear tape, but instead coordination and dexterity in the fingers and hands. Figure 1-18, A, shows a strip of tape being held firmly between the thumb and first finger of each hand and being torn by a quick scissor-like movement of the wrists in opposite directions.

Figure 1-18, (B) shows a method whereby the taper holds the tape in the preferred hand with the thumb pressing its outer edge. The other hand grasps the loose end between the thumb and first finger, and again a quick scissor-like movement of the wrists in opposite directions is employed.

Tearing Tape

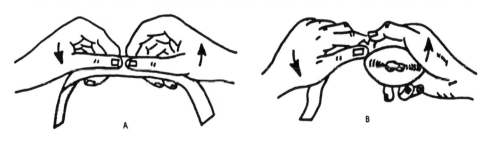

A   B

Fig. 1-18

ATHLETIC INJURIES
AND ASSESSMENT

ATHLETIC INJURIES

An **athletic injury** is defined as a disruption in tissue continuity that results from athletic or sports-related activity, causing a cessation of participation or restriction of usual activity. This definition implies that an athletic injury is more than the aches and pains that may accompany but not interfere with athletic participation. There is an almost infinite array of possibilities in the spectrum of athletic injuries, ranging from minor problems to severe and potentially lethal types of trauma.

Athletic injuries result from the application of forces or stresses in excess of the body's or body part's ability to adapt. The manner and location by which these excess forces or stresses ae applied to the body, better known as the **mechanism of injury**, determines the exact nature and extent of the injury and the tissues involved. These forces or stresses may be applied (1) instantaneously, resulting in an **acute traumatic injury**, or (2) over a considerable period of time, resulting in a **chronic overuse syndrome**. Traumatic injuries such as sprains, strains, and contusions are common to athletic activity, particularly during contact sports. Overuse syndromes such as tendinitis, bursitis, stress fractures, and shin splints are becoming much more common in athletic activity because of the increasing intensity of training and conditioning programs. As a group, the overuse injuries occur more often in athletic activity requiring specific repetitive movements.

Athletic injuries are grouped into two main classifications, depending on the integrity of the skin: (1) the **exposed** injuries, and (2) the **unexposed** injuries. Exposed, or open, injuries are those that disrupt the continuity of the skin. Unexposed, or closed, injuries are those that are internal and do not break the skin. An athlete can suffer an injury in both classifications simultaneously; for example, an external blow resulting in a laceration and contusion.

EXPOSED ATHLETIC INJURIES

Open wounds are normally caused by physical trauma and may range from a simple scratch to a large, deep, freely bleeding laceration. Table 2-1 outlines the five common types of open wounds. It is important to remember that an open wound may only be surface evidence of a more severe and often "hidden" athletic injury. Most open or exposed athletic injuries are minor in severity and do not result in significant hemorrhaging or loss of tissue. However, any bleeding must be controlled before a complete evaluation of the wound itself or of the possible involvement of deeper anatomic structures. The application of direct pressure over the site of bleeding, preferably with a sterile dressing (Figure 2-1), should be sufficient to control the hemorrhaging of most open wounds. The risk of infection is usually a greater concern in treating an exposed wound than the amount of bleeding.

Types of Open Wounds

Type	Cause	Characteristics	Care
Abrasion	Fall Scraping or rubbing of skin away	Superficial Little bleeding, oozing, or weeping	Clean Remove debris Antiseptic Sterile dressing
Laceration	Wound made by tearing	Jagged edges May bleed freely Contusion & tearing Often leaves scar	Control bleeding Clean Suture if required Inspect daily
Incision	Cut by sharp object	Smooth edges Freely bleeding	Control bleeding Clean Suture if required Inspect daily
Puncture	Penetration by sharp object	Small opening Minimal bleeding	Clean Referral Inspect daily
Avulsion	Tearing loose flap of skin	Completely loose Hanging as a flap May bleed freely	Control bleeding Clean Save avulsed piece Referral

Table 2-1

Application of Direct Pressure to Control Bleeding

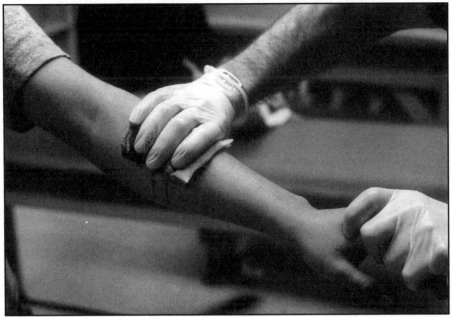

Fig. 2-1

You must also remember to protect yourself whenever working with open wounds or when any bodily fluids are present. The athlete may have a systemic infection or the open lesion may contain some type of pathogenic microorganism. Personal health demands attention to infection barriers and proper hygiene. Hands should be washed thoroughly before and after contact. Disposable gloves should be worn anytime you are working with body fluids. Any equipment or instruments used in conjunction with an open wound should be thoroughly cleaned and disinfected before and after each use. An infection control program begins with our own personal health.

Abrasions

Abrasions occur when the epidermis and a portion of the dermis is scraped or rubbed away (Figure 2-2). This type of injury is very common in athletic activity and is usually caused by falling on a firm or rough surface. Athletes commonly refer to abrasions as "mat burns,"

Abrasion

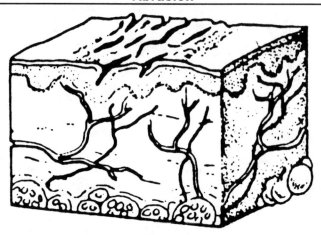

Fig. 2-2

"floor burns," or "cinder burns," depending on the surface that caused them. A reddish, irregular surface appearance gives rise to the descriptive name "strawberry." The bleeding associated with abrasions is usually limited to blood oozing from underlying injured capillaries. Although these injuries may be painful, the primary concern is that of infection. The abraded area will often contain contaminants such as bits of dirt, debris, or bacteria embedded in the injured tissue.

An abrasion must be cleaned thoroughly. Soap and water will work well, but the area should be cleaned with an antibacterial scrub. Care must be taken to remove all foreign material from the wound. Depending on the circumstances of injury, you may have to use a soft brush to clean the area thoroughly. A traditional method of caring for an abrasion is to apply an antiseptic to the area after the wound has been cleaned and covered with a sterile, nonadhesive dressing. An ointment dressing is often applied when the abrasion is in the vicinity of a joint so that a scab does not form and be continually reopened during activity.

The contemporary treatment of abrasions involves a variety of self-adherent occlusive, hydrocolloid dressings. These dressings, applied after the abrasion has been thoroughly cleaned, do not allow a scab to form by keeping the wound moist. This method has been shown to allow reepithelialization to occur faster than abrasions exposed to air. Occlusive dressings have also been found to assist in relieving the pain associated with abrasions. Abrasions should be evaluated and cared for daily with either of these treatment routines.

> An abrasion should be referred to a physician for any of the following reasons:
>
> 1. It is impossible to remove all the foreign material by washing the wound.
> 2. The area surrounding the abrasion becomes inflamed and infected a few days after the injury.
> 3. There is doubt about the status of the abrasion.

Lacerations

Lacerations are wounds or cuts made by tearing and are common in athletics (Figure 2-3). These injuries are usually the result of some type of direct blow to the skin and are especially common over bony prominences. The skin may be stretched and actually torn apart. Lacerations are often described as a combination of contusion and tear. The edges of a laceration are usually jagged or irregular, and at least some surrounding tissue damage occurs in most laceration injuries. The severity of lacerations can range from a very small crack in the skin to a large, deep wound with associated damage to surrounding and deeper structures. The nature and severity of bleeding associated with lacerations is quite variable.

Laceration

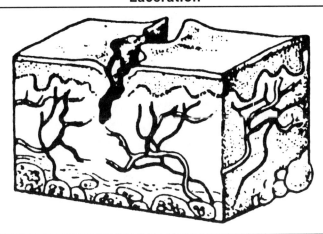

Fig. 2-3

Incisions

Incisions are wounds caused by cutting with some type of sharp object, such as a knife (Figure 2-4). The edges of an incision are smooth and cleanly cut, with little damage to surrounding tissue. Occasionally, an incised wound will be deep and damage blood vessels, muscles, tendons, or nerves well below the skin surface. Fortunately, severe incision wounds rarely occur as a result of athletic activity.

Incision

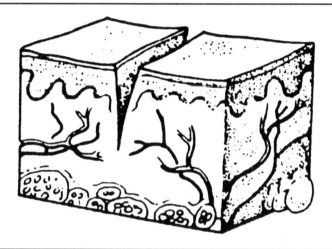

Fig. 2-4

The initial care for incisions is essentially the same as for lacerations. Once bleeding has been controlled, carefully clean and inspect the wound. Is there any foreign material embedded in the wound? How deep is the wound? Was the mechanism of injury sufficient to cause other injuries in addition to the open wound?

Athletic trainers and coaches often must differentiate between lacerations and incisions that are "playable" and those that are not. Generally athletes will continue to play with smaller (less than 1 inch), superficial, and uncomplicated lacerations after the wound has been sufficiently treated. After the game the athlete can be referred to medical care. Occasionally, all that is necessary is to close the edges of the cut or tear with adhesive strips, such as butterfly closures (Figure 2-5) or Steri-Strips, and apply a sterile dressing. In many cases, however, sutures are indicated. Because of activity required during athletics,

Using Butterfly Closures

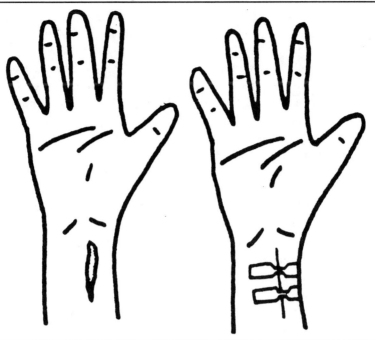

Fig. 2-5

sutures are more frequently recommended for athletes than nonathletes. Lacerations and incisions also need to be protected against additional trauma and stretching when the athlete returns to participation. The wound should be inspected daily for any signs of infection or further trauma.

The athlete should be referred to a physician for any of the following reasons:

1. The wound may need sutures for adequate closure (more than 1/2-inch length and 1/8-inch depth)
2. There is foreign material embedded in the wound which cannot be removed
3. Bleeding persists despite all efforts to control it
4. The wound is on the face or another part of the body where scar tissue will be noticeable after healing
5. The surrounding area becomes inflamed or infected
6. There is doubt about how the laceration or incision should be treated

Puncture Wounds

Puncture wounds occur as a result of direct penetration of the skin by a pointed object (Figure 2-6). The opening may be quite small, with little or no bleeding. The penetrating object may, however, damage underlying structures and carry contaminants into the body. One of the first considerations in caring for a puncture is to determine the depth of penetration and the possibility of underlying damage. Only if the puncture is very minor and the penetrating object small, with little depth of penetration, are you justified in simply cleaning the wound and observing for signs of infection. The majority of puncture wounds should be cleansed and promptly referred to a physician. Large items that remain imbedded should be left in place until a physician can remove them. A tetanus toxoid booster is often indicted with puncture wounds. Punctures are not common in athletics but should be properly cared for when they occur. These wounds should be inspected frequently for signs of infection.

Puncture

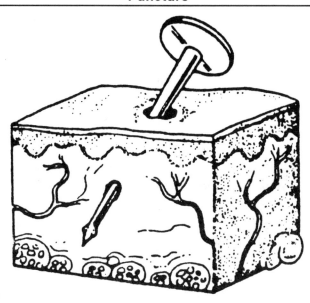

Fig. 2-6

Avulsions

An avulsion is the tearing away of part of a structure. When referring to an open wound, an avulsion is the tearing loose of a piece of skin, which may be torn completely free or remain partially attached, hanging as a flap (Figure 2-7). There may or may not be much bleeding. If an avulsed piece of skin or tissue of significant size is torn completely free of the athlete, it should be saved and transported with the athlete to a medical facility. The avulsed portion should be wrapped in sterile gauze and kept moist and cool. Occasionally, significant portions of avulsed tissue may be successfully reattached. When the avulsed part remains attached, the flap of skin should be placed back in its normal position before bandaging and referral. Small flaps of skin, especially in highly vascular body areas such as the scalp and face, may remain viable and heal if replaced.

Avulsion

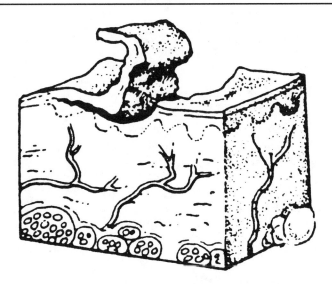

Fig. 2-7

UNEXPOSED ATHLETIC INJURIES

Unexposed, or closed, athletic injuries are internal, with no associated disruption or break in the continuity of the skin. Unexposed injuries can result in massive bleeding and significant damage to underlying structures, with little or no visible signs at the skin surface. Structures commonly involved in athletic injuries of this type include soft tissues such as muscles, tendons, blood vessels, and ligaments. Unexposed athletic injuries also involve such structures as bones, nerves, and internal (visceral) organs and their linings. The common unexposed athletic injuries are classified into contusions, strains, sprains, dislocations, and simple fractures (Table 2-2).

Types of Closed Wounds

Type	Cause	Characteristics	Care
Contusion (bruise)	Direct blow	Hematoma Ecchymosis Local tenderness	ICER Symptomatic care Protect
Strain	Overstretching Overstressing Violent contraction Strength imbalance	1°-Stretching Some discomfort No disability 2°-Tearing of fibers Pain Some instability 3°-Complete rupture Disability Deficit	ICER Symptomatic care Minimal support ICER Symptomatic care Support ICER Referral
Sprain	Joint forced in abnormal direction	1°-Stretching Some discomfort No instability 2°-Tearing of ligament Pain Some instability Swelling 3°-Complete rupture Instability Swelling	ICER Symptomatic care Minimal support ICER Protection Support ICER Referral
Dislocation	Joint forced beyond anatomical limits	Deformity Pain Loss of function	Cold Immobilization Referral
Fracture	Direct blow Indirect blow Twisting force Repetitive stress	Pain Crepitation Deformity Loss of function Guarding	Cold Immobilization Referral

Table 2-2

Contusions

A contusion is a bruise and is among the most common type of injury occurring in athletic activity (Figure 2-8). Contusions usually result from a direct blow or impact being delivered to some part of the body, which causes damage to underlying blood vessels. The resulting bleeding into the skin or subcutaneous tissues may produce symptoms that range from very minor areas of discoloration to extremely large, debilitating masses. The collection of blood that forms at the site of a contusion is called a **hematoma**. As the blood leaks into the subcutaneous tissues, it will often cause a black and blue discoloration known as **ecchymosis**. In addition to the swelling, a bruise usually results in an area of local tenderness.

Contusion

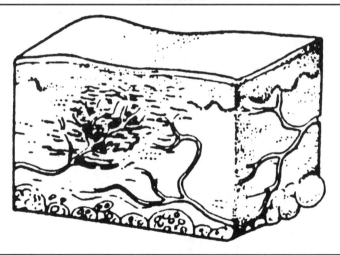

Fig. 2-8

The tissues involved in a contusion, as well as the amount of damage and bleeding, will depend on the force of the impact, the size and the shape of the object causing the bruise, and the part of the body receiving the blow. For example, a blow to a large muscular area such as the thigh will result in damage or bruising to the muscles. The involved muscles respond by protective muscle spasms, causing a deceased excursion of the muscle fibers and a reduced range of motion (ROM) at the associated joints.

The objective of the initial treatment of contusions is to control the bleeding by means of ice, compression, and elevation. Heat and activity during this initial period may encourage or promote bleeding and should be avoided. Once bleeding has stopped and the athlete exhibits a near normal range of motion without a significant increase in pain, activity may be resumed. The level of activity is increased according to the athlete's tolerance until participation is at the level demanded by the sport. During recovery the athlete should be protected from reinjury by padding the bruised area and by avoiding excessive activity, which may aggravate the injured tissues.

Strains

Strains are injuries involving the musculotendinous unit and may involve the muscle, tendon, and the junction between the two as well as their attachments to bone (Figure 2-9). Strains or pulls can be caused by a variety of mechanisms, such as overstretching, overstressing, a violent contraction against heavy resistance, a strength imbalance between agonists and antagonists, or an abnormal muscular con-

Strains

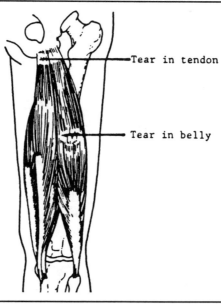

Tear in tendon

Tear in belly

Fig. 2-9

traction. These injuries are generally dynamic; that is, there is no out-side intervention and the athlete injures himself or herself. The por-tion of the musculotendinous unit that is damaged depends on which component is the weakest link in the chain at the moment of injury. Generally, in younger athletes whose growth centers have not closed, the muscles and tendons are stronger. With these athletes the attach-ments to the bone may fail and actually avulse a piece of bone with the tendon or separate at the epiphyseal, or growth line (epiphyseal frac-ture). In older athletes, the tendons and musculotendinous junctions become the weaker links and are more susceptible to injury.

Strains are graded into three groups by level of severity. Each is determined by the amount of damage to the fibers of the musculotendinous unit. The definitions, and the signs and symptoms delineating each grade of severity, are as follows.

A **mild strain (first degree)** involves stretching and a minimal amount of tearing of the involved tissues. Although there is some dis-comfort during function after a mild strain, there is generally little or no disability. An athlete has normal or near-normal range of motion and experiences only insignificant loss in strength. Athletes with these in-juries require only minimal protection and support, such as an elastic wrap, to continue participation. Many times an athlete will continue ac-tivity and not report mild strains unless symptoms become more severe.

A **moderate strain (second degree)** involves a significant tear-ing of fibers, although at least some continuity of the musculotendinous unit remains. A few fibers may be torn, or the majority of the fibers in a given unit may be damaged. An athlete may complete a workout or activity in pain after suffering a moderate strain and then experience disability later that day or the next morning. The second-degree strain is the most common type of strain. Signs and symptoms accompany-ing moderate strains include varying degrees of pain, swelling, loss of strength, and loss of flexibility. The athlete may hear or feel a snap at the time the tissue tears. An area of point tenderness is evident on pal-pation, as is local pain expressed during active, resistive, or stretching movements. Occasionally a palpable gap, or deficit, is evident immedi-ately after the injury. The athlete should be treated symptomatically and returned to activity as tolerated. The time required for return to complete activity varies from a few days to several weeks after a mod-erate strain. Athletes normally require protection and support for the injured area when they return to activity.

A **severe strain (third degree)** involves complete destruction of the hear or feel a snap as the tissue ruptures. Usually there will be an associated palpable, and many times visible, gap at the site of injury. The muscle may bunch up because of spasmodic contractions. The athlete will experience a significant weakness and loss of function as a result of the injury. Severe strains should be treated initially with cold, compression, and elevation and then referred to a physician for further diagnosis and treatment.

> Strains should be referred to a physician for any of the following reasons:
> 1. A visible or palpable gap is noted.
> 2. Muscle fibers bunch as the result of spasmodic contractions and lack attachment of one extremity to a fixed point.
> 3. The athlete demonstrates a significant weakness and loss of function.
> 4. There is doubt about the status of the strain.

Acute musculotendinous strains resulting from athletic activity occur most frequently in the lower extremities. Treatment is aimed at restoring flexibility and strength. A period of complete inactivity will often result in a shortened, atrophied muscle that must be gradually stretched and strengthened to its normal state before full activity can be resumed. Severe strains therefore require repeated evaluations in order to return the athlete to full activity as quickly as possible.

Chronic strains can result from abuse or overuse of the musculotendinous unit. The most frequent mechanisms of injury involve workloads that are too stressful for the musculotendinous unit to withstand. Training and conditioning programs are designed to strengthen this contractile unit gradually, so that it is able to withstand progressively heavier work loads and thereby avoid strains. Chronic inflammation of a muscle may result if an athlete trains too intensely, performs specific repetitive movements over a considerable period of time, or continues to use an injured area. Any area of the musculotendinous unit can become irritated and inflamed, such as the muscle (myositis), the tendon (tendinitis), the musculotendinous junction, the tendon and its protective synovial sheath (tenosynovitis) or the tendinous attachment to bone. Although each of these chronic over-use syndromes involves a different area of the contractile unit, they require basically the same treatment. Treatment procedures normally include rest, local heat, anti-inflammatory medication, and protection against continued aggravation. Most treatment programs require a modification of activity, or perhaps complete rest, which may be difficult and frustrating for both the athlete and the coach. After the cessation of symptoms, the athlete must resume activity gradually and progress within tolerable limits to avoid recurrence of the injury.

Sprains

A sprain is an injury involving a ligament. Ligaments are basically inelastic and designed to prevent abnormal motion at a joint. Whenever a joint is forced to move in an abnormal direction, ligaments are stressed (Figure 2-10). If the ligament is forced beyond its limit, damage will occur at the weakest link in the ligament. The damage may be within the ligament itself or at one of its attachments. The severity of damage depends on the amount and duration of the abnormal force.

Sprain

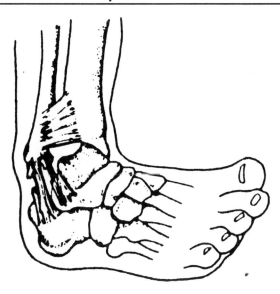

Fig. 2-10

Hinge joints, those designed to function in only one direction or plane, are the most frequently sprained. Sprains may occur dynamically; for example, the injury may be self-inflicted during twisting or turning activity. Most sprains, however, involve some outside intervention, such as getting hit on the side of the leg or landing on someone or something in the wrong way.

Ligament sprains are among the more common injuries in athletics. They also are graded into three levels of severity, determined by the amount of ligament damaged.

A **mild sprain (first degree)** involves minor stretching or tearing, with minimal disruption in the continuity of the ligament. Although there may be some discomfort during function, there is little or no disability. The athlete will have no instability or abnormal motion of the joint during passive stress tests. The ligament is not weakened significantly, and the treatment is symptomatic. An athlete may continue activity and not even report a mild sprain.

A **moderate sprain (second degree)** involves a tearing of ligament fibers and a partial break in the continuity of this non-contractile structure. Like second-degree strains, moderate sprains include the widest range of severity and are the type most common. Moderate sprains are the most difficult to assess. Long experience and refined assessment skills are needed to determine with accuracy the amount of damage sustained by a ligament in a second-degree sprain.

Moderate sprains include varying degrees of pain, swelling, and instability. The athlete may hear or feel a snapping sensation as well as sense something giving way at the time of the injury. The torn fibers of the injured ligament will produce local pain and instability. The amount of instability will depend on the number of ligament fibers torn or ruptured. Aslong as some of the ligament remains intact, the passive stress test will normally have an end point, or a perceived limit to abnormal motion.

The goal when caring for moderate sprains is primarily to protect the injured ligament during the healing process. Protection is mandatory to keep the damaged fibers immobile and close together in order to promote efficient repair. If injured ligaments are subjected to repeated stresses and reinjury during this healing process, they may heal in a lengthened and weakened state, resulting in an unstable joint. In most cases protection must be provided by external means, such as a cast, brace, splint, or tape. Once the healing ligament is moderately strong, the surrounding muscles can be rehabilitated to assist in support and to provide protection. Remember, ligaments heal by developing scar tissue, which takes a minimum of 6 weeks to develop and may take 6 months or longer to mature and provide maximum strength.

A **severe sprain (third degree)** involves a complete rupture and break in the continuity of the ligament. This may involve the ligament pulling loose a piece of bone at its point of attachment, causing an avulsion fracture. The athlete frequently hears or feels the ligament snap and has the sensation of the joint giving way in this type of injury. The athlete may or may not have pain initially with a completely torn or severed ligament. Passive stressing will produce significant instability and no end point of motion.

Athletes suspected of having severe sprains should be treated with routine initial procedures, splinted, and referred to a physician for further diagnosis and surgical repair if necessary. Frequently surgical repair is required to reposition the ligament ends to ensure healing at or near normal length.

Sprains should be referred to a physician for any of the following reasons:

1. Significant instability is demonstrated by passive stress tests.
2. Significant joint effusion occurs within a few hours after the injury. **Effusion** is swelling within the joint space.
3. There is doubt about the status of the sprain

Dislocations

A dislocation is the displacement of contiguous surfaces of bones composing a joint (Figure 2-11). This type of injury results from forces, usually external, that cause the joint to go beyond its normal anatomical limits. This may occur as a result of excessive force or from force in an abnormal direction. When there is an incomplete displacement of the bone ends, the injury is called an incomplete dislocation or subluxation. Because ligaments function to prevent displacement or abnormal motion at joints, all sprains result in some degree of **subluxation**. A complete dislocation, or **luxation**, occurs when there is a complete separation of the bone ends. A dislocation will either remain displaced after injury or reduce spontaneously and move back

Dislocation

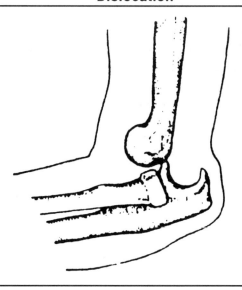

Fig. 2-11

into place. It may be difficult to evaluate exactly what happened unless the athlete can document the dislocation. Many times the athlete is aware that the bones are out of place, andcan relate the position of the joint when it was dislocated. Dislocations may be accompanied by avulsion fractures, which can be verified by radiographs, and by torn ligaments, resulting in moderate to severe sprains.

Joints that are designed to function in one direction or plane, such as hinge joints, are those more severely injured when dislocated. For example, when the ankle, knee, or elbow are dislocated, there is normally a significant amount of damage to surrounding structures. Damage to nerves and blood vessels is also more likely. On the other hand, when the shoulder, which has a great range of motion and few restrictions, is dislocated, long-term complications and damage to nerves and blood vessels are not as common.

Dislocations that remain displaced are generally easy to recognize. Deformity is almost always apparent. Occasionally you may have to palpate and compare body contours with the uninjured extremity to reveal minimal deformity. Dislocations also cause a significant amount of pain as well as loss of limb function. The objective of treatment is reduction of the dislocation by a physician. Initially, splint or support the injured joint to prevent any further damage. All suspected dislocations should be referred to a physician for radiographs and further evaluation.

Treatment for dislocations, once they are reduced, depends on the joint involved, but essentially is the same as that for severe sprains. Surgical intervention is sometimes required, and the injured ligaments must be supported and protected throughout the healing process. Unprotected joints may heal with increased laxity in the ligaments, making the joints more vulnerable to subsequent subluxations and total dislocations.

Fractures

A fracture is a disruption in the continuity of bone and can range in severity from a simple crack to the severe shattering of a bone with multiple fragments. Fractures are unique injuries in that they heal with the same type of tissue (bone) that was injured and can thus regain their preinjured strength. Bones can be fractured in several ways. A direct blow may cause a break at the point of impact, such as an athlete getting kicked in the lateral aspect of the leg, resulting in a fractured fibula. An indirect blow may cause a fracture away from the point of impact, such as an athlete landing on his or her hand and breaking one of the bones of the upper extremity. Severe twisting forces, such as turning and cutting maneuvers, may also cause a fracture. As previously described, severe sprains or strains may result in avulsion fractures.

Prolonged repetitive activity or chronic overuse can lead to another type of fracture, **stress fracture**, sometimes called fatigue fracture. These types of fractures occur over a considerable period of time and without history of an acute traumatic episode. Stress fractures are generally incomplete fractures and seldom result in separation of bone fragments. Many times the initial plain-film radiographs will be negative, and the stress fracture will not be confirmed until the appearance of new periosteal bone formation is recognized on follow-up radiographs two or three weeks later. The actual fracture line may never appear on radiographs. Suspect a stress fracture when an athlete reports painful stress and tenderness over a bony area without any specific trauma but is involved in an activity with repetitive stress. If symptoms persist, repeated radiographs or a bone scan may be required to obtain a definitive diagnosis.

Fractures are divided into two major classifications according to involvement of the overlying skin. Fractures that do not break the skin are called **closed fractures**, whereas fractures that are associated with a tear of the skin are **open fractures** (Figure 2-12). Open fractures may be caused by a broken bone end tearing the skin, or by a direct blow that lacerates the skin at the time of fracture. These are generally the more serious type of fractures because of the additional possibilities of infection and external bleeding.

Fractures

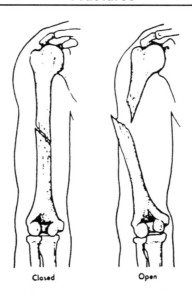

Closed   Open

Fig. 2-12

There are many signs and symptoms that may assist you in recognizing a fracture. The primary symptom is pain localized at the fracture site that remains consistent with motion, palpation, or stress maneuvers. The athlete may report the sound or sensation of something breaking or snapping. The athlete may also experience a grating or grinding sound (**crepitation**), which is caused by the bone ends rubbing against each other during any type of movement. There may be an obvious deformity or irregularity of the involved area such as swelling, protrusion, or shortening of a limb. With a compound fracture, a broken bone end may or may not be protruding through the open wound. There may be a loss of function or disability associated with a fracture. However, a loss of function does not always accompany a fracture and it is a myth to believe, "If the injured part can be moved, it's not broken." The detection of any of these signs and symptoms deserves additional assessment procedures and referral to medical assistance for further diagnosis and radiographs. Athletes may also demonstrate false motion or abnormal movement in an area, which is commonly called a false joint. However, in the presence of the above signs and symptoms there is little need to demonstrate false motion. In the absence of signs and symptoms indicating a fracture, more vigorous procedures should be applied to evaluate the bony integrity. A forceful levering both longitudinally and cross-wise to the bone should be performed before pronouncing any such injury free of fracture. You must maintain a high index of suspicion and never allow an athlete to return to activity with an injury that suggests a fracture. Similarly, you must not decide any suspected fracture is safe from aggravation by continued athlete activity without further diagnosis.

The treatment for suspected fractures is that of protection for the injured area so that no further damage occurs because of improper handling or movement. This is normally accomplished by splinting the injured area. Remember to immobilize the joint above and below a fracture site to avoid movement to the bone fragments. If there is an open wound associated with the fracture, control the bleeding and apply a sterile dressing before splinting the area. Treat for shock if necessary. Feel for a pulse distal to major fractures to ensure circulation is adequate. Whenever circulation is jeopardized, a medical emergency exists and the injured athlete must be transported to a medical facility immediately.

ATHLETIC INJURY ASSESSMENT

The athletic injury assessment process is a necessary and extremely important skill for anyone who shares the responsibility for the medical care of athletes. It consists of an ordered sequence of procedures used to evaluate the nature, site, and severity of an athletic injury. When an injury occurs, early, accurate evaluation is important in developing an effective treatment and rehabilitation program.

The assessment process can be divided into two major parts: (1) the **primary survey** and (2) the **secondary survey**. Each survey is important and should be considered with each injury.

PRIMARY SURVEY

The primary survey is that portion of the evaluation concerned with life support mechanisms of Airway, Breathing, and Circulation. These are usually referred to as the ABC's of life support. The probability that life-threatening situations will arise as a result of athletic injuries is minimal; however, everyone involved in athletics must be aware that the potential for serious injury does exist. Life-threatening conditions must be recognized immediately and dealt with effectively to prevent needless loss of life.

With most athletic injuries, the primary survey is completed easily and quickly. For example, if an athlete is conscious and talking, you can assume he or she is breathing and has a pulse. If the athlete is lying motionless and unconscious, you must then evaluate his or her breathing and pulse. Rarely, this portion of the assessment process requires that you open the airway and initiate CPR maneuvers. However, everyone involved with athletics should know those important life-saving skills.

SECONDARY SURVEY

The secondary survey is that portion of the assessment that examines the athlete is an attempt to recognize and evaluate all injuries or related conditions. This usually comprises the largest portion of the total athletic injury assessment process. The secondary survey can be divided into three main areas: **History, Observation**, and **Physical Examination** (Figure 2-13). An accurate assessment of an athletic injury often times depends upon a factual and reliable history; studious and diligent observations; and a careful and complete physical examination. The remainder of this unit will discuss various concerns and procedures for each of these important segments of an athletic injury assessment. Of course, not all the procedures discussed under each area of the secondary survey will be carried out with each athletic injury. The nature, type, and severity of the injury will determine the evalua-

Basic Steps of the Secondary Survey

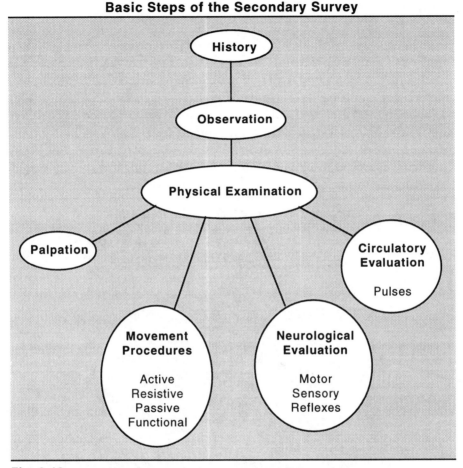

Fig. 2-13

tive techniques used. Every coach will at some time be faced with an athletic injury requiring very few assessment skills; for example, a fractured arm with the bone protruding through the skin. With this type of an injury, immediate first aid and referral skills are the primary concern. Except in these types of obvious injuries, then you should always initiate and conduct some type of a sequential assessment process. Short cuts in evaluating athletic injuries should be avoided, as they increase the risk of overlooking or missing important information. Coaches having the responsibility for athletic injuries must continue to improve and refine their assessment skills.

History

Obtaining an accurate history of an injury is one of the most important steps in the secondary survey portion of the total athletic injury assessment process. Taking a history involves finding out as much information as possible about the actual injury and the circumstances surrounding its occurrence. This is accomplished by talking with the injured athlete or others who have either witnessed or observed the injury (Fig. 2-14). Information gained in a thorough history can provide important clues in determining which structures may be injured and which assessment techniques will be appropriate as you continue the examination.

Obtaining a History from an Injured Athlete

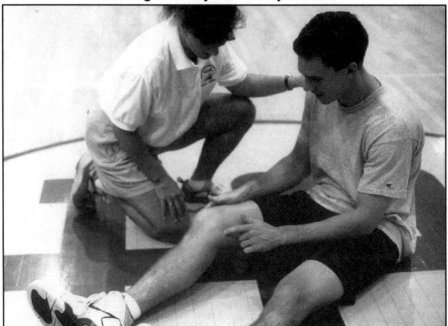

Fig. 2-14

Athletic injuries can happen almost anywhere and anytime during activity. They basically appear in two ways; (1) suddenly, such as those caused by trauma, and (2) gradually, such as the overuse syndromes that develop over a period of time. The direction taken when obtaining the history depends on the nature of the injury and how it occurred.

Injuries that Appear Suddenly

The history of a sudden traumatic injury is usually easy to obtain. Normally you would talk with the injured athlete. Since this type of injury is frequently witnessed, perhaps others can provide useful information to help in completing the history. In some cases an athlete may not report the injury at the time it occurs or when the symptoms initially appear. Then, in addition to the history of the injury, you must find out what, if anything, has occurred since the injury happened. Specific questions required to elicit necessary information will vary, depending on the nature of the injury in question. Piecing together the complete history requires time, skill, patience, and thoroughness.

Injuries that Appear Gradually

Accurate assessment of athletic injuries that develop over a period of time, such as chronic injuries and overuse syndromes, requires a very detailed history. Sometimes the onset of the symptoms may be insidious, and the athlete will have few recollections of any injury or stress. The symptoms usually begin as a mild and sporadic ache and gradually become more painful and continuous. You must attempt to gain a much information as possible related to the injury. Did the symptoms appear suddenly or did they come on gradually? What has the athlete been able to do since the symptoms first appeared? Inquire about functional capabilities such as the ability to walk, climb stairs, twist, throw, or whatever activity is involved with the body area injured. What aggravates the injured area? Is it relieved by rest? Injuries that appear gradually may be caused by any of a number of factors, such as errors in training, inappropriate or improperly fitted equipment, playing surfaces, structural abnormalities, poor flexibility, or poor conditioning. The history must take into consideration all of these factors.

There are several important factors to remember in attempting to gain a comprehensive history. Each of these factors involves the development and use of communication skills. To gain an accurate history of the injury, you must communicate with the injured athlete if at all possible. The athlete is the only person who has experienced the injury and knows exactly how it feels. Of course, there will be times when it will be impossible to talk to the injured athlete; for example, if he or she is unconscious or unresponsive for any reason. When this occurs, you must question other athletes or persons who might have witnessed the injury. Attempt to gain as much information as possible from whomever observed the injury or has knowledge of important factors associated with its occurrence.

There are other considerations to keep in mind as you attempt to talk with an injured athlete. Immediately after an injury, the athlete may not feel like talking. He or she may be in pain and frightened or panicky. Perhaps the last thing the athlete wants to do at that time is carry on a conversation about the injury. You should appreciate that every athlete responds differently to an injury. Some explain their injury in great detail, whereas others volunteer little if any information. Some athletes try to minimize their injury, whereas others try to maximize it. In addition, some persons become very emotional when in pain or under stress. These circumstances often complicate the assessment process and underscore the need to communicate with an injured athlete in a calm and reassuring manner. Make every attempt to relax the athlete so that he or she will be able to discuss the injury and respond to questions.

When speaking with the athlete, keep the questions simple. Most athletes are not interested in carrying on lengthy conversations after sustaining an injury. Ask only one question at a time and get the answer before proceeding on to the next.

Each injury and each injured athlete is unique. You must develop interview or questioning skills that can be applied in a wide variety of situations. Clarify the information being gathered and ask questions that will elicit further essential information. Ask relevant, nonleading questions of an injured athlete. Examples of leading questions are "Did you turn your ankle under?" and "Does it hurt right here?" It is much easier for an athlete in pain to answer "yes" to such questions than to describe the injury in detail. If you lead the athlete with your questions, you may actually develop a false impression of the injury. Let the athlete describe the injury and tell you what happened.

As the athlete explains how the injury occurred, it is important to listen attentively to what he or she is saying. Many clues as to the structures injured, as well as severity of injury, can be gained by listening to the athlete's description of the injury. It is easy to make assumptions about an injury, especially if the injury was witnessed. If the athlete says he or she heard and felt a popping or cracking sensation and believes something is broken, it must be assumed correct until proven otherwise. Give the athlete the benefit of the doubt, even if it appears that he or she is overreacting to the injury. Do not start the assessment with your mind made up about the injury. Each new injury must be evaluated separately. Begin with a complete history, and allow the athlete to describe the injury and spell out in detail exactly what happened. The importance of being a good listener cannot be overemphasized.

In communicating with an injured athlete, determine the **primary complaint** early in the assessment process. Where does it hurt? What type of injury has the athlete suffered? Attempt to find out the exact **mechanism of injury**. How and when did the injury occur? Did the athlete fall or was there a twist? Did the athlete hear or feel anything? Attempt to recreate in your mind the mechanism of injury and visualize the position of the body when the injury occurred. It is important to have a clear conception of the mechanism of injury.

Attempt to locate the areas of **pain**. It is helpful if the athlete can point to where the pain is. Notice how he or she points to the painful area. Is the pain localized or is it spread over a large body area? Be as exact as possible in determining anatomic location. Is the pain around a joint, along a bone, or in a muscular area?

Inquire about the **functional abilities** of the injured athlete. Athletes may be able to perform with minimal amounts of pain or only occasional pain. Is there pain only during function or movement? Is the pain intensified by movement or activity? Is the pain constant or intermittent? Seek specific information concerning the nature of pain associated with athletic injuries.

In addition to the pain, ask the athlete to describe any **other symptoms** associated with the injury in as much detail as possible. Is the athlete experiencing any numbness, tingling, weakness, or burning sensations? Is reference made to any type of grinding or grating sensations (crepitation). Did the athlete experience any abnormal sounds or sensations at the time of the injury? Does the athlete feel any tightness, tension, or swelling associated with the injury?

Talking with an athlete will also assist in assessing his or her **level of consciousness**. For example, is the athlete alert and responsive or confused and disoriented? It is important to evaluate the athlete's level of consciousness and establish a neurologic baseline early in the assessment process, especially when the injury involves the head.

Knowledge of past injuries or problems can greatly help in assessing the nature of current injuries. Inquire about any **previous in-**

juries to the affected part or surrounding body area. If there was a previous injury, probe for additional details. What type of injury? How long was the recovery period? Was the recovery complete? What kind of treatment and rehabilitation programs were followed? All of this information can be helpful in assessing current injuries. Also attempt to find out about any other **pre-existing medical conditions** that may have a relationship to the injury, or any **medications** the athlete may be taking.

The more relevant information that can be gained from a history, the more accurately the injury can be evaluated. Do not overlook the importance of obtaining the history even though you witnessed the injury and believe you know exactly what is injured and how it occurred.

Observation

The next step of the secondary survey, observation, begins when you first see the injured athlete and continues until the assessment process is completed. Much information can be gained through observation skills. Several important points should be remembered in observing an injured athlete. Begin by quickly surveying the entire scene. Notice the **position** of the athlete. Did you observe the **mechanism of injury**. Was there any apparatus or equipment associated with the injury? Look for any obvious **bleeding, deformity, swelling, discoloration**, or any **other signs** of injury. Note general body alignment and posture of the athlete. Is the athlete holding a body part or grasping some body area? If the athlete is moving around, observe his or her **functional abilities**. Is the athlete using the injured part or protecting it? Is he or she limping?

After a general survey of the injury scene, carefully inspect the injured area and assess the results of the athletic injury (Figure 2-15). This is often accomplished in conjunction with the history-taking process. Watch closely as the athlete describes the injury. What is the position of the injured part? Be alert for any **signs of trauma**, such as abrasions or contusions, that may indicate the mechanism of injury. Some athletes try to disguise or minimize the extent of their injury. Observing the athlete's face and eyes as he or she describes the injury may give further clues as to the extent of pain. More pain may be reflected in the athlete's face than he or she is willing to admit.

Inspecting an Injured Area

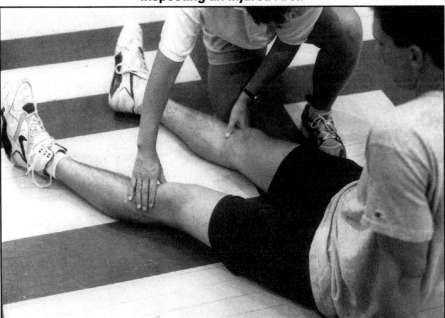

Fig. 2-15

When inspecting an injury, clothing and equipment that may obscure the area should be removed. Consider the athletes modesty in removing clothing and equipment. If possible, adequate exposure should permit visualization of the area above and below the injury. Do not limit your examination solely to the area of injury. You should always compare the injured body part to the contralateral uninjured part and note any obvious differences. However, you must be aware of any abnormalities in the uninjured body part caused by such things as congenital conditions or previous injuries.

Physical Examinaiton

The third phase of the secondary survey involves the selective use of a variety of assessment procedures and maneuvers designed to further locate and evaluate the integrity of the structures involved in the injury. These procedures can be broken down into the following areas: **palpation, movements procedures, neurological evaluations,** and **circulatory evaluations.** Each area can be important and informative. However, not all procedures will be necessary with every athletic injury. Which evaluative procedures or maneuvers are used and in what sequence will depend upon the athletic injury. For example, for an athlete with a suspected spine injury, the motor and sensory function evaluations would become extremely important and be performed very early in the assessment process. Following is a basic description of each area of the physical examination. Specific tests and procedures to evaluate various injuries are explained throughout this manual.

Palpation

Palpation means to touch and feel the injured area. After the history and observation steps, you can gain additional physical information concerning the injury by carefully palpating the affected body area (Figure 2-16).

Palpating an Injured Area

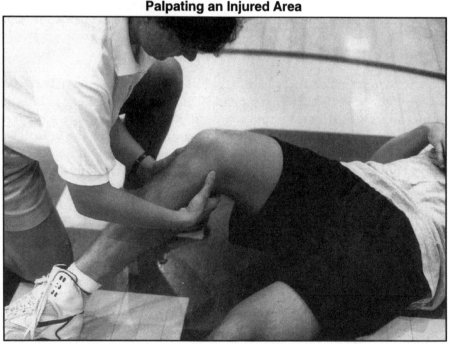

Fig. 2-16

There are several important points to remember as you prepare to palpate an injured athlete. Palpation procedures should begin in a tender manner to avoid unnecessary pain. If you cause the athlete unnecessary pain, he or she may become tense and uncooperative, making palpation assessment of the injury more difficult, if not impossible. To accurately palpate an injured area it should be as relaxed as possible. Treating the athlete gently helps demonstrate your concern and helps establish confidence and cooperation. The intensity or pressure used with each palpation maneuver can then be increased, depending upon the athlete's tolerance and the severity of the injury. It is also a good practice to begin palpating away from the injury site to encourage the athlete's cooperation and confidence. In addition, by doing this you are not as likely to become so involved with the obvious injury that you overlook another, less apparent injury.

It is important that you visualize what structures are under your fingers. Are you feeling approximately where ligaments should be? Are you feeling an isolated tendon or a musculotendinous junction? Are you palpating predominately muscular tissue or bone? To visualize the structures that are being palpated, you must have an understanding of the underlying anatomy. It may be helpful to look at anatomic charts or drawings to verify underlying anatomy and show them to the injured athlete to help him or her understand the injury. Remember to also compare contralateral areas.

Important information can be gained by careful palpation procedures. **Pain** is one of the most obvious and consistent symptoms of injury. Use of palpation techniques to localize pain is extremely useful in assessing athletic injuries. It is especially important to locate areas that are most painful to touch. These are called areas of point tenderness. Regardless of the anatomic structures involved, **point tenderness** is usually found at the site of injury. This location of point tenderness, along with knowledge of underlying anatomic structures can provide important clues in evaluating the site and nature of an injury.

Another physical sign that can be recognized by palpation is **swelling**. Swelling or edema may be localized at the injury site or diffused over a larger area. Swelling may result from bleeding caused by trauma or by accumulation of pus or tissue fluid as a result of some inflammatory process. As a rule of thumb, the amount of swelling is generally related to the severity of injury. There are cases, however, in which serious injuries produce very limited swelling, and minor injuries cause severe and extensive swelling or edema.

Additional information gained during palpation may be related to the **temperature** and **surface moisture** of the skin. Normal skin is moderately warm and dry. In palpating the site of an injury, any indication of an increase in skin temperature would suggest the occurrence of an inflammatory process. A decrease in skin temperature may be felt in areas of inadequate circulation. In addition, various combinations of skin color, temperature, texture, and moisture can assist in identification of generalized conditions such as shock and problems associated with body temperature regulation.

Muscle spasms may also be recognized while palpating an injured area. This is a body defense mechanism designed to protect an injured area from further trauma. When an injury occurs, the surrounding muscles often involuntarily contract or become tight as the body attempts to splint or brace the injured area. The area surrounding an injury may then feel tense or tight as you palpate the area. Remember to instruct the athlete to relax the injured area as much as possible before beginning palpation procedures.

Deformity is another physical sign that may be discovered during palpation. The cause may be a fracture, dislocation, or the tearing of soft tissue such as ligament, muscle or tendon. Deformity may be quite obvious and easily seen on observation, or it may be very discreet and only recognized after carefully palpation of the injured area. If there is any question regarding what the normal contour of the area should be, the corresponding uninjured side should be palpated as a basis for comparison.

Crepitation is a grating, grinding, or sticking sensation that may be produced by various conditions. When crepitation is associated with athletic injuries, it is commonly caused by the broken ends of a bone rubbing together or the thickening of synovial or bursal fluids and membranes. An athlete may describe a grinding sensation on movement of an injured part, and you may feel crepitus as you palpate the injured area.

Movement Procedures

Up to this point in the assessment process, the injured athlete does not have to move or be moved. If necessary, history, observation, and palpation can be completed with the athlete remaining in the original position he or she is in immediately after injury. Movement procedures, however, do involve some movement of a body part or the athlete. However, should a serious injury be suspected, it is not necessary to perform this step of the assessment process, and appropriate emergency measures should be initiated.

Movement procedures involve selective use of some type of manipulation or stress to the injured body area. These procedures are employed in an attempt to further locate and define the structures involved in the injury, as well as to evaluate the integrity of affected tissues. Information gained in this way is extremely valuable and usually cannot be obtained in any other manner. A complete and detailed evaluation of an athletic injury is often not possible unless the injury is subjected to some movement or stress.

There are several important factors to remember as you prepare to stress an injured area. Movement procedures should not be applied to an injured area until history, observation, and palpation have been completed. You must have an idea as to the nature of the injury before you attempt to move the affected body part. For example, you would not attempt to stress an injured area when you suspect a dislocation or fracture. In addition to the information gained, completion of these three steps in the secondary survey serves another useful purpose. It provides the time necessary to calm and relax the athlete before manipulation and stress testing begins.

It is important that you explain what you are going to do and elicit cooperation from the athlete before beginning any stress tests. It is extremely difficult to use movement maneuvers effectively in assessment procedures if the injured athlete is tense and unable to relax. A mutual sense of trust between the athlete and coach is essential to gain accurate information from the assessment. In addition to development of trust, the ability to communicate effectively is especially important during this step of the evaluation process.

Applying stress to an injured area will undoubtedly cause some additional pain. However, these procedures should not cause unnecessary pain, or you will most likely lose the cooperation of the injured player. Any stress applied to the athlete should begin slowly and gently to minimize pain and protective muscle spasms. In a painful injury, it is a good practice to begin these maneuvers on the uninjured side. This will help lessen apprehensions and prepare the player for procedures that will be carried out on the injured side. This can also give you information necessary to compare the injured to the uninjured side.

Although there are many procedures for applying stress to an injured area, they can be divided into four basic types of maneuvers or movements: (1) active, (2) resistive, (3) passive, and (4) functional. Seldom is it necessary to subject an injury to tests from all four groups. Information gained during the first three steps in the assessment process will enable you to select the most appropriate procedures.

Active Movements. Active movements are those that can be initiated and completed by the athlete without assistance of any kind. Such movements are usually the least stressful. To initiate this type of maneuver the athlete is asked to move the injured part as directed by the athletic trainer. Active motion is used to evaluate the athlete's willingness and ability to move the injured area. Active movements also assess the integrity of contractile and related tissues such as muscles and tendons and their junctions, attachments, integration, and control by the nervous system. Noncontractile tissues, such as joint capsules, ligaments, bursae, cartilage, and nerves, will also have some stress applied to them as the result of active motion. Note which movements, if any, cause pain and the amount and quality of pain that results. Does the movement increase the intensity of the pain? Where and when in the movement does the pain occur? Is there any restriction or limitation in the active motion?

Another important factor that can be evaluated with active motion is the range of motion (ROM) of surrounding joints. For example, an athlete may be asked to actively move an injured extremity through the pain-free ROM. Active motion will indicate the athlete's ability and willingness to perform the movements requested as well as the ROM possible. Pain will normally limit active motion so that additional injury to damaged structures does not occur as a result of the assessment process. Note the limits of active motion and if necessary compare it to the ROM of the uninjured side.

Resistive movements. Resistance may be applied against active motion to further evaluate the integrity of the contractile tissues. Whenever a muscle or tendon injury is suspected or indicated, resistive movements can assist in identifying specific tender areas. Usually resistance is applied manually (Figure 2-17). Manual resistance can be applied throughout the ROM or isometrically in various positions in the range. Resistance applied isometrically (static contraction) helps rule out non-contractile tissue involvement and stresses primarily the contractile tissues. Low initial resistance against movement is gradu-

Manual Resistance Applied Against an Injured Body Part

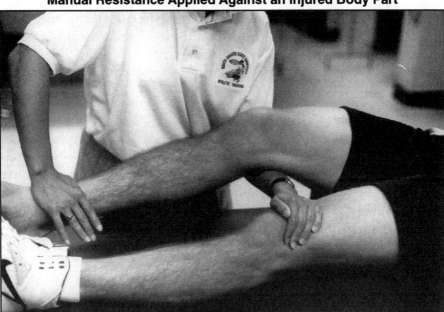

Fig. 2-17

ally increased, depending on the athlete's tolerance. The ability of the athlete to tolerate increasing resistance loads can reveal a great deal about the extent of injury involving the contractile tissues. Note the site of pain at any specific point throughout the resisted ROM.

Resistive movements are also used to evaluate the strength of a body part. During the acute stages of an athletic injury, pain will normally limit an accurate evaluation of muscular strength. However, on repeated assessments used to determine when an injured athlete is ready to return to activity, manual muscle testing can be very beneficial in evaluating muscular strength. Manual muscle testing is normally performed throughout a full ROM for each muscle or group of muscles. The athlete is positioned in such a way that isolates the muscle or group of muscles being tested and allows movement through the full ROM. Substitution by muscles other than those being tested can usually be eliminated by careful positioning. Manual resistance is then applied throughout the movement by the athlete or the athlete offers resistance to the movement performed by the athletic trainer. Those same resistive movements are usually performed on the contralateral or uninjured side for a comparison of strength. It is often necessary to carefully repeat manual muscle tests, comparing the strength to the normal side, because weaknesses can be subtle. Note weaknesses and differences in strength.

Passive movements. Passive movements are procedures performed completely by someone else and are the most difficult stress procedures to perform and evaluate (Figure 2-18). The athlete is asked to relax the injured area so that the effects of conscious control and muscular effort can be eliminated. Great care must be exercised in performing passive movements because the potential to cause additional pain or injury is much greater than during active and resistive movements. Initially, these stress procedures must be performed very gently and slowly to avoid causing unnecessary pain and muscle spasms. The intensity of the procedures can then be increased, depending on the athlete's tolerance and the severity of injury.

Passive movements are used to evaluate the integrity of noncontractile tissues such as bones, joint capsules, ligaments, and bursae. There are numerous passive tests designed to analyze and lo-

Passive Stress Applied to a Joint

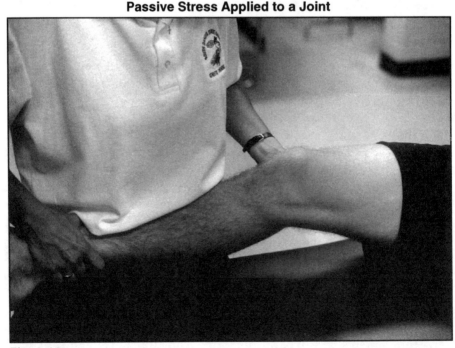

Fig. 2-18

cate any instability, pain, or crepitation present as the result of an injury. For example, each ligament about an injured joint should be stressed to check for pain and instability. The extent of instability or laxity must be recognized and noted to properly determine the severity of injury. These passive tests are often designed to reproduce the mechanism of injury. Some specific passive procedures used to locate pain and instability in athletic injuries are described and illustrated throughout the remainder of this manual.

Functional movements. Functional movements are a series of active movements or activities the athlete performs that simulate the type of activity required in a particular sport. These tests can be used during the initial assessment of an athletic injury, but are most often used to determine if recovery is complete and if the athlete is ready to return to full participation or activity. The athlete is asked to perform specific movements necessary or required in his or her sport. In most cases the first functional movements are designed to generate relatively little stress. Stress intensity is then increased for subsequent movements until the extent of injury is determined or full recovery is apparent. For example, the athlete with an injured leg may be asked to begin jogging; if that does not cause any pain or problems, the athlete may progress to running and then jumping or cutting activities, depending on the sport.

Functional testing should always precede the return of the athlete to full activity. An athlete who has full strength and no pain or instability on active or passive stress tests must also demonstrate the ability to perform any activities required of his or her sport before returning to full participation.

Neurological Evaluations

There are many neurological examinations that may accompany an assessment process. Coaches should posses a basic knowledge of neurologic examinations of the level of consciousness, sensory functions, and motor functions.

Sensory functions. Assessing the neurologic status of sensory functions is accomplished by applying various stimuli to specific areas of the skin that are innervated by particular sensory nerves. Testing for altered sensations is usually completed quickly after an athletic injury. Run a relaxed hand or fingers over the entire skin surface to be tested on the injured side, as well as the corresponding uninjured side. Does the athlete feel any difference in sensations between the two sides of the body? If an area of altered sensations is found, localize the area or determine the boundaries. More specific tests can also be performed, such as testing for sensitivity to light touch or pain sensation. To assess touch use a cotton swab, soft brush, or lightly scratch the skin's surface and note the athlete's response. To test for pain, apply the sharp and dull points of a pin or instrument to the skin and note whether the athlete correctly perceives the stimulus. Again, compare sensations to the uninjured side. Testing for sensory function is especially important in assessing head and spinal injuries but should also be used after significant injuries involving the extremities. If distal sensations are normal, it may be assumed the peripheral nerve is intact.

Motor function. Evaluation of motor function is carried out by asking the athlete to move the injured part as has been previously discussed with active (ROM) and resistive movements (manual muscle testing). When a spinal injury is suspected, ask the athlete to carefully move his or her fingers or toes. Then proceed to the larger joints. If the athlete has normal motion in the extremities, proceed to check the speed and strength of movements. When a nerve injury is suspected or to evaluate the integrity of a specific spinal nerve, check the muscle or group of muscles supplied by that nerve.

Circulatory Evaluations

The obvious importance of assessing if an athlete has adequate circulation was previously discussed under the primary survey. It is also important to evaluate the circulatory status in an extremity following an athletic injury to that area (Figure 2-19). After a fracture or dislocation it is especially important to palpate for a pulse distal to the injury to determine if the extremity has sufficient circulation. If no pulses are found distal to an injury, a medical emergency may exist, and appropriate care and referral measures should be initiated immediately.

Evaluating the Circulation of An Injured Extremity

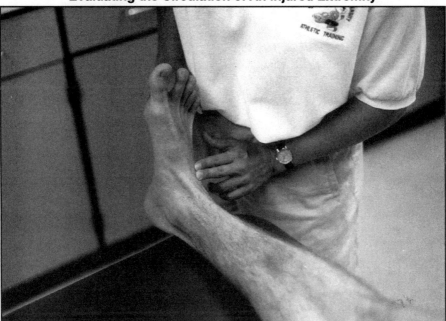

Fig. 2-19

Summary

Figure 2-20 outlines the athletic injury assessment process in a checklist form. Obviously, not all athletic injuries require as complete and systematic a survey as outlined. Coaches must learn to select the appropriate evaluation procedures based on the injured body part and the findings obtained throughout the assessment process. To become skilled in athletic injury assessment, a person must be well versed in both functional anatomy and the procedures used during the evaluation process.

Athletic Injury Assessment Checklist

Primary survey

☐ **Airway**   ☐ **Breathing**   ☐ **Circulation**

Secondary Survey

☐ **History**
- ☐ primary complaint
- ☐ mechanism of injury
- ☐ areas of pain
- ☐ functional abilities
- ☐ other associated symptoms
- ☐ level of consciousness
- ☐ previous injuries
- ☐ pre-existing conditions and medications

☐ **Observation**
- ☐ bleeding
- ☐ deformity
- ☐ swelling
- ☐ discoloration
- ☐ signs of trauma
- ☐ skin appearance
- ☐ expressions denoting pain
- ☐ symmetry

☐ **Physical Examination**
Palpation
- ☐ point tenderness
- ☐ pain

- ☐ swelling
- ☐ deformity
- ☐ crepitation
- ☐ muscle spasms
- ☐ skin temperature

Movement Procedures
- ☐ active movements
  - ☐ ROM
  - ☐ pain
- ☐ resistive movements
  - ☐ pain
  - ☐ weakness
- ☐ passive movements
  - ☐ instability
  - ☐ pain
  - ☐ crepitation
- ☐ functional movements
  - ☐ functional abilities

Neurological Evaluations
- ☐ sensory functions
- ☐ motor functions
- ☐ reflexes

Circulatory evaluations
- ☐ pulses

Fig. 2-20

INJURIES TO THE LOWER EXTREMITIES

The lower extremities are complex functioning units extremely important to athletic activity. Because of its great utilization and diversified functions, this area of the body is continually subjected to many traumatic stresses. The lower extremities are involved in more injury-related conditions or problems than any other area of the body. This unit will briefly discuss the more common athletic injuries which may occur to the lower extremities as well as describe taping procedures which are frequently used.

FOOT

Our feet form the foundation of our body. During athletic activity our feet support our body weight in a myriad of positions and adapt to a multitude of surfaces and contours. As such, our feet continually bear the brunt of physical stresses and rapidly changing forces thrust on them from all directions and are frequently involved in athletic injuries.

Each foot is composed of 26 bones: seven tarsals, five metatarsals, and 14 phalanges (Figure 3-1). Like the fingers, there are three phalanges for each digit except the big toe, which has two. The phalanges are designated as proximal, middle, and distal. Normally the tarsals and metatarsals play the major role in the functioning of the foot as a supporting structure, with the phalanges being relatively unimportant. In the hand, where manipulation rather than support is the main function, the reverse is true.

The interphalangeal joints are hinge joints and permit only flexion and extension. The metatarsophalangeal joints permit flexion, extension, and some abduction and adduction. The intertarsal, tarsometatarsal, and intermetatarsal joints permit only gliding movements. The subtalar joint is the point of articulation between the talus and the calcaneus. This is also a gliding joint. The motions of inver-

Bones of the Foot and Ankle

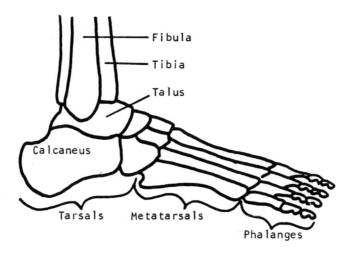

Fig. 3-1

sion and eversion occur simultaneously at these gliding joints. A limited range of inversion and eversion are extremely important to the athlete and enables the body to move sideways over the foot while the foot itself remains fixed.

     Pronation of the foot is a combination of abduction, dorsiflexion, and eversion. These motions take place in the tarsal joints and especially the subtalar joint. Some pronation is normal, but excessive pronation, or hyperpronation during weight bearing, is a common condition found in athletes who exhibit overuse problems of the feet and legs. In fact, this defect is considered to be the most common cause of chronic overuse injuries in runners. The hyperpronated foot is considered to be a very flexible foot with excessive motion at the subtalar joint. When the foot pronates, the weight line falls to the medial side of the foot, the medial longitudinal arch depresses, and the toes tend to be directed outward. Other common signs of a pronated foot include an inward tilting of the heel, causing a medial curving of the Achilles tendon and a more pronounced medial malleolus. These deviations result in an abnormal relationship between the talus, calcaneus, and tarsal articulations with each foot strike, and a variety of chronic overuse syndromes in the foot, leg, and knee can result.

The amount of pronation of the foot can range from quite mild to very severe. The mildly pronated foot may present fatigue and pain in the arch as well as a generalized postural fatigue, especially with running activities. The moderately pronated foot has increased mobility and poorer shock-absorbing qualities at heel strike. The toes are more unstable, and the intrinsic muscles fatigue more quickly. There is a higher incidence of overuse injuries such as plantar fascial strains, heel bruises, calcaneal spurs, bursitis, tendinitis, and stress fractures. The severely pronated foot is a hypermobile flatfoot with very little longitudinal arch visible during weight bearing. The athlete with hyperpronated feet are often fitted with orthotics to improve foot mechanics.

A less common foot type is one that does not pronate sufficiently. This is a foot with a high longitudinal arch and limited tarsal motion. This is called a **cavus foot** and is considered to be an inflexible foot that does not adequately absorb shock or easily adapt to various surfaces. The cavus foot is usually associated with heavy callus formation on the ball of the foot or heel caused by additional stresses placed on these areas. Clawing of the toes and pain along the bottom of the foot or under the metatarsal heads is typical. In addition, the cavus foot transmits increased shock to the ankle, leg, knee, thigh, hip, or back, creating an increased incidence of overuse injuries.

The cavus foot can range from a flexible foot to one that is very rigid. The flexible cavus foot has a high arch when it is not bearing weight and has somewhat limited shock-absorbing qualities. As the cavus foot becomes more rigid, the high arch and claw toes become less flexible. The arch will flatten only mildly and the claw toes do not straighten completely with weight bearing. This foot has more callus build-up and frequent pain under the metatarsal heads because increased abnormal stresses transmitted to this area are common. The rigid cavus foot is the most difficult foot to manage. This foot has a very high longitudinal arch and clawed toes at rest and when bearing weight. It has a tight plantar fascia, and painful calluses usually develop under the metatarsal heads. The rigid cavus foot does not absorb shock well, adapts to surfaces very poorly, and is inadequately suited for athletic activity. Athletes with this type of foot are more susceptible to sprained ankles, Achilles tendon problems, arch conditions, stress fractures, and a variety of overuse injuries.

ARCHES

The bones of the foot are held together in such a way as to form springy, lengthwise (**longitudinal**) and crosswise (**transverse**) arches. The arches are formed by the placement of the metatarsals and tarsals and held in place by strong ligaments and tendons from muscles originating in the leg. These arches provide a highly stable and resilient base to bear the body's weight, absorb the shocks associated with activity, and provide space under the foot for blood vessels, nerves, and muscles to pass.

Longitudinal Arch

The longitudinal arch (Figure 3-2) is made up of the medial and lateral portions of the foot and extends from behind the metatarsal heads back to the heel. As previously discussed, some athletes have a very high rigid longitudinal arch which absorbs shock poorly and is not conducive to repetitive activity. More commonly athletes may have a very mobile foot in which the longitudinal arch may flatten too much during weight bearing. In this type of foot there is a higher incidence of overuse injuries. There are several methods of taping for support of a sprained, weakened, or painful longitudinal arch.

Longitudinal Arch

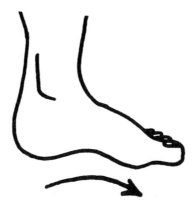

Fig. 3-2

Figure 3-3 illustrates a commonly used taping procedure for the longitudinal arch called the figure eight. The foot should be placed in a relaxed position. Start with an anchor strip (#1) around the metatarsal heads. Using 3/4"-1" tape, the second strip starts on either side of the ball of the foot, continues diagonally across the arch, encircling the heel, and ending on the opposite side (#2). This forms an "X" in the middle of the arch. These strips are repeated (usually 3-4 times) to provide enough support for the arch. The ends of tape are locked by encircling the foot with another 3-4 strips of tape as shown in B.

Figure Eight Taping

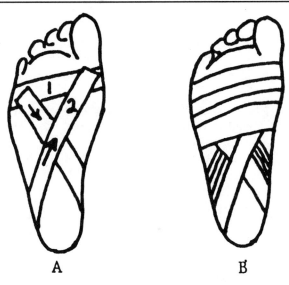

A   B

Fig. 3-3

Another popular method of supporting the longitudinal arch is called the LowDye technique (Figure 3-4). Apply an anchor strip from the head of the fifth metatarsal, behind the heel to the head of the first metatarsal (#1). Remember to keep this strip low on the foot. Now apply bridging strips beginning on the lateral anchor, circle under the plantar surface and finish on the medial side (#2-#6). Lock these encir-cling strips with another piece of tape similar to the initial anchor. Repeat this entire procedure a second time and lock it down with a couple of strips encircling the forefoot (C).

Low Dye Taping

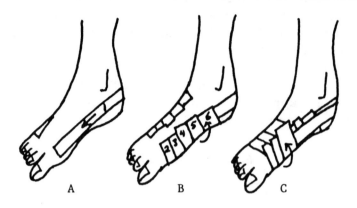

Fig. 3-4

Figure 3-5 shows a method of taping a half-moon shaped vinyl foam rubber pad into the longitudinal arch area. Taping should start on the outside of the foot, continue under the arch, come up on the inside and encircle the foot (B).

Taping Pad in Longitudinal Arch

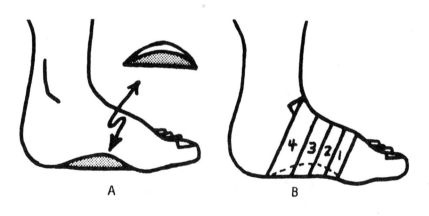

Fig. 3-5

Transverse Arch

The transverse arch is perpendicular to the length of the foot (Figure 3-6). Essentially, there are a series of transverse arches across the plantar surface of the foot. Occasionally athletes will complain of pain just behind the metatarsal heads, an area which is referred to as the metatarsal arch. Figure 3-7 illustrates a method of supporting this arch using an "egg" shaped vinyl foam rubber or felt pad placed just behind the metatarsal heads and held on by encircling strips of tape around the foot.

Transverse Arch	Taping Pad in Transverse Arch

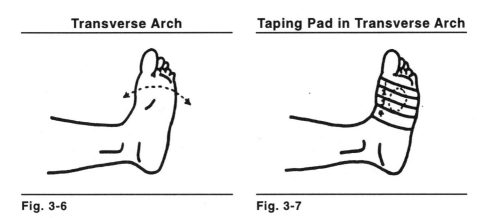

Fig. 3-6   **Fig. 3-7**

FOOT CONDITIONS AND INJURIES

Contusions

Contusions about the foot resulting from various types of direct impacts are common in athletics. Although painful initially, these injuries are generally not serious. However, contusions to the plantar, or weight bearing surface of the foot, can be particularly bothersome and handicapping. This injury is normally caused by direct trauma such as repeated pounding on hard surfaces, stepping on an object, or a faulty spike or cleat. The subcutaneous tissue between the bones of the foot and the thick plantar skin becomes bruised and inflamed. The area may become quite painful and disabling during weight bearing and athletic activity. A common site for this type of contusion is the heel, also called a **stone bruise**.

A heel cup or a pad of vinyl foam rubber can be very helpful in protecting a bruised heel. This area can also be taped for protection by alternating strips of 3/4"-1" tape to produce a basketweave effect over the entire heel area (Figure 3-8). The strips should be put on fairly tight and locked by a strip of tape going completely around the leg (B).

Taping Heel

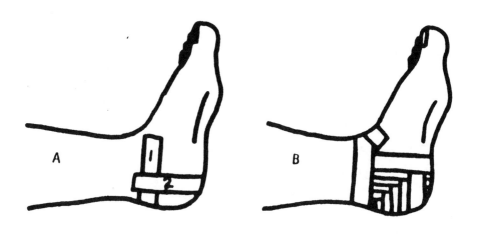

Fig. 3-8

Strains

Strains involving the muscles and tendons about the foot can result from overuse or violent stresses. These injuries usually cause cramping or fatigue of the involved muscles. These symptoms normally subside when activity is reduced or discontinued. A common strain of the foot occurs to the plantar fascia, which is a strong band of connective tissue that is one of the primary supports for the longitudinal arch. A strain to this structure is called plantar fasciitis. Support for this type of injury was previously discussed and illustrated along with the longitudinal arch.

Sprains

Injuries involving the ligaments or capsules surrounding the joints of the foot are common in athletics. The most common site for a sprain in the foot is the metatarsophalangeal joint of the great toe. This is sometimes referred to as a **turf toe** because it frequently occurs on artificial turf. This type of an injury can become very handicapping as the great toe is very important in weight bearing and must bear the brunt of every step. Symptomatically, sprains about the toes will be tender at the site of injury with an increase in pain on reproduction of the stress that caused the injury. There are normally varying amounts of swelling, stiffness, and soreness surrounding the articulations. Depending on the amount of ligamentous damage, there may be varying amounts of instability associated with the injury. If instability is recognized, the athlete should be referred to medical assistance.

Figure 3-9 shows a method of taping for a sprained or malaligned great toe. Using 1/2"-3/4" tape, place an anchor behind or around the metatarsal heads (#1). Run strips of tape around the metatarsophalangeal joint in a figure eight pattern (A). The pull of the tape can be in either direction depending on the injury. It is much easier to apply the tape by placing it between the toes to start. Apply figure eight strips until the athlete tells you that the painful motion is reduced

Taping Great Toe

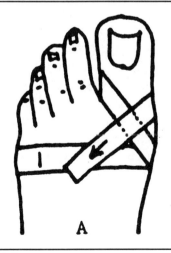
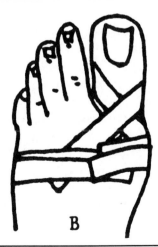

Fig. 3-9

sufficiently for continuation of activity. Make certain the strips of tape are not put on too tightly to impair circulation. Lock the strips by encircling the ball of the foot with tape as shown in B. This taping procedure illustrated is to prevent or limit flexion of the great toe. To limit extension, the tape should cross on the plantar surface of the joint.

The midfoot is composed of the navicular, cuboid, and three cuneiform bones. The midtarsal and tarsometatarsal joints are supported by a strong ligamentous system that is not injured often. However, midfoot sprains can result from severe twisting mechanisms or forceful direct trauma that causes a subluxation of the involved tarsals or metatarsals. These sprains produce tenderness at the site of injury, and quite often weight bearing is extremely painful. This type of injury can be very painful and prevent an athlete from normal activity for a considerable length of time. Midfoot sprains are supported in the same manner as the longitudinal arch described previously.

Blisters

Blisters commonly occur on the feet, especially during the early season, when the skin of the feet is soft and not accustomed to athletic activity. Over a period of time the skin will accommodate the friction, becoming tougher and much less likely to blister. Blisters are usually caused by friction or shearing forces. As a result, there is a separation of the outer layer of the skin (epidermis) from the inner layer (dermis) and fluid accumulates in this area. The fluid is normally a clear exudate that has escaped from tiny blood vessels in the area. If the shearing force actually ruptures a blood vessel, the blister may be filled with blood. Occasionally a blister will become infected and filled with pus. The friction or shearing forces are enhanced by such things as poor-fitting or faulty equipment (especially shoes), participation on extremely hard surfaces, continued repetitive activity, or activity requiring frequent starting, stopping, and changing of direction. Athletes will normally feel a blister developing by detecting a "hot spot".

There are two general methods of treating blisters: conservative and radical. The step-by-step procedure for both methods is listed on the following page and illustrated in Figure 3-10.

Treatment of Blisters

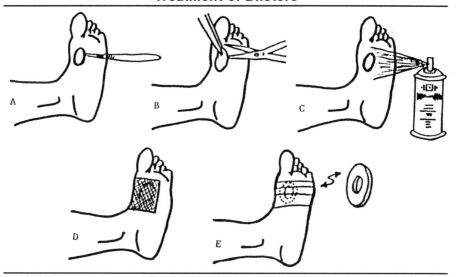

Fig. 3-10

Step 1.   The blister and surrounding area should be cleansed with soap and water or alcohol.

Step 2.   The base of the blister should be punctured with a sterile scalpel, scissors, or needle (A).
Conservative approach. The fluid is normally drained but · the loose skin is not removed. Check the area daily for any signs of infection. After a few days, the loose dead skin may be trimmed away. A thick layer of skin covering a deep blister may reattach and not have to be removed. The conservative approach is usually preferred when there is little danger of tearing or aggravating the blister through activity.
Radical approach. All loose skin is cut away from the blister (B). This approach is preferred when the skin is already torn and aggravated by activity.

Step 3.   Apply an antiseptic to the area (C).

Step 4.   Apply an ointment dressing to the exposed area, especially the first few days when the tissue is sore and raw (D).

Step 5.   The blister should be protected during activity by either a donut-shaped pad placed over the area (E) or the use of a product such as second skin. Both of these techniques can also be used when just walking around if the area is particularly tender.

A donut is used to relieve pressure on painful areas. The felt pad is usually about 1/4" thick with the hole slightly larger than the lesion. Donuts can also be used to protect warts, abrasions, excess calluses, bone spurs, cuts, or other painful irritations during activity. It is very important that a donut be well secured in place with tape so that it will not slip and cause undue pressure and pain.

Athlete's Foot

Athlete's foot is a very common fungal infection. This condition is characterized by redness, scaling, cracking, and itching on the skin surface of the feet, most commonly between the toes. These organisms thrive in a dark, warm, moist environment and can be transmitted from one athlete to another. Sweating, heat, and physical activity contribute to the growth of fungi. Athlete's foot is best treated by drying thoroughly after a shower, applying a fungicide, and wearing clean, white socks.

Calluses

Calluses are a thickening of the outer layer of skin which develop from constant friction, pressure, or irritation. Excess callus formation can become painful and disabling as the mass becomes hard and inelastic. The most frequent sites of excess callus formation are under the metatarsal heads, the outer edge of the heel, and the inner edge of the big toe. Treatment consists of preventing the excess callus accumulation and protecting the involved area. Once excess callus tissue has formed, it should be softened and trimmed to the level of the surrounding skin periodically to prevent further problems. If painful, a donut may help relieve the pressure.

ANKLE

The ankle joint is the linkage between the foot and leg. This hinge joint, which is one of the more frequently injured in the body, allows only plantar flexion and dorsiflexion. The ankle is often described as a three-sided box-like or mortise joint. The top of the box is the articulating surface of the tibia. The sides are formed by the medial and lateral malleoli. This socket articulates with the talus below. The **medial malleolus** is the distal end of the tibia and the **lateral malleolus** is the distal end of the fibula. These bony landmarks serve as attachments for the supporting ligaments of the ankle and can be easily palpated. The ankle joint is designed for weight bearing and has great bony and ligamentous strength.

The bones that compose the ankle are held together by a strong fibrous capsule that is attached to the articular margins of the tibia and fibula above and to the talus below. In addition to the capsule, the distal ends of the tibia and fibula are tightly bound to each other by ligaments at the distal tibiofibular articulation just above the ankle. This distal tibiofibular articulation is a fibrous type of joint, called a **syndesmosis**. Stability of the distal tibiofibular syndesmosis is maintained by the anterior and posterior tibiofibular ligaments and the interosseous membrane. Occasionally athletes will suffer syndesmosis sprains of the ankle.

The capsule of the ankle is subdivided into four ligaments: (1) anterior tibiofibular, (2) posterior tibiofibular, (3) medial (deltoid), and (4) lateral. These ligaments are identified on Figures 3-11 and 3-12. The deltoid or medial ligament is triangular, thick and very strong. In extreme or forced eversion of the foot, the deltoid may tear or fracture the medial malleolus. The lateral ligament complex is composed of three separate ligaments: (1) anterior talofibular, (2) posterior talofibular, and (3) calcaneofibular. These three ligaments are not as strong as the deltoid and are injured much more frequently. Most ankle injuries involve these ligaments.

Lateral Ankle	Medial Ankle

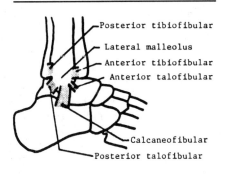

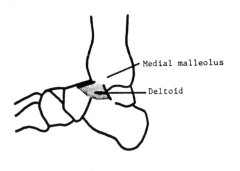

Fig. 3-11

Fig. 3-12

Ankle Sprains

Ankle sprains are among the most common athletic injuries. The frequency results from the anatomical structure, the weight-bearing function, and the violent forces applied to this joint during athletic activity. As previously discussed, the talus fits into a mortise formed by the distal ends of the tibia and fibula. The talus is narrower posteriorly than anteriorly. This anatomical fact explains the slight looseness or increased amount of motion of the ankle joint in plantar flexion. The talus fits more snugly into the mortise during dorsiflexion. The ankle joint is designed to function as a hinge joint permitting only dorsal and plantar flexion. Ankle injuries occur when this joint is forced to the extremes of motion or in an abnormal direction.

The most common mechanism of injury occurs when the ankle is forced into inversion. Because of the shorter medial malleolus, inversion occurs more readily than eversion. Therefore, the ankle has a normal tendency to go into inversion when striking an irregular surface, such as coming down on another athlete's foot. Most athletic activity also predisposes an athlete to inversion types of stresses since most cutting and turning maneuvers are initiated by the foot opposite the direction of the turn which can force the foot into inversion and place stress on the lateral ligaments.

The opposite mechanism of injury, forced eversion, occurs less frequently during athletic activity. This can occur when the leg is hit laterally with the foot fixed. Because the lateral malleolus is as long as the talus is high, it is very difficult for the lower end of the fibula to act as a fulcrum during this type of an injury. This fact, along with the strength of the medial ligaments, explains why isolated injuries to the deltoid ligament are seldom seen. Sprains to the medial side of the ankle are often severe and involve additional structures such as a fractured fibula.

Syndesmosis sprains of the ankle are uncommon injuries. This injury occurs as the tibia and fibula are forced apart injuring the ligaments that bind these bones together. Often the mechanism causing a syndesmosis ankle sprain is forced dorsiflexion. As the foot is forced into dorsiflexion, the broad part of the talus is located firmly between the malleoli and may force the bones apart, thus injuring the ligaments of the distal tibiofibular joint. A similar injury can result from forced rotation of the leg with the foot firmly fixed. In these cases the shape of the talus acts as a fulcrum forcing the tibia and fibula apart. It is important to differentiate the syndesmosis sprain from the more common lateral ligament sprain because this sprain often causes more disabling symptoms and has a prolonged recovery time. Symptoms include point tenderness and swelling localized over the anterior and posterior tibiofibular ligaments. There may be some pain over the medial malleolus and/or the interosseous area. The athlete will often prefer to walk on his or her toes and complain of an inability to "push off."

Significant ankle sprains are almost always accompanied by immediate pain and difficulty in bearing weight. Local tenderness will be exhibited over the ligaments involved, and there may or may not be initial swelling or restriction of motion. It is important to evaluate the severity of the sprain before swelling develops and motion becomes restricted.

As with any evaluation, begin with an accurate history and review the forces or stresses associated with the injury. Localize the painful area and then attempt to recognize an unstable ankle. This is accomplished by the use of passive tests. Compare the amount of inversion and eversion of both ankles by stabilizing the leg with one hand and passively moving the foot with the other (Figure 3-13). Alternately invert and evert both feet in an attempt to locate any pain or abnormal movement associated with these movements. Pain along the course of one of the lateral ligaments that increases with passive inversion suggests that the ligament has been sprained. It may be very difficult to assess the degree of abnormal movement with this test unless there is an obvious instability.

Passively Inverting Foot

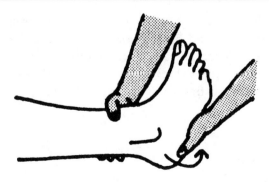

Fig. 3-13

Another procedure that should always be performed on a suspected ankle sprain is the **drawer test**. This tests the integrity of the anterior talofibular ligament, which is the most commonly injured at the ankle. This test is performed on a relaxed leg by stabilizing the leg with one hand and grasping the heel with the other. The calcaneus is then lifted forward while the tibia is kept steady (Figure 3-14). If the ligament is intact, there should be no movement of the foot in relation to the leg. If, however, the ligament is ruptured, the drawer test will be positive and the talus will slide forward from under the tibia. Whenever this test is positive, the athlete should be referred to a physician.

Drawer Test for Ankle

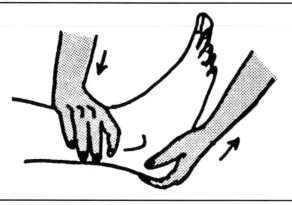

Fig. 3-14

ANKLE SUPPORT

Due to the frequency of ankle sprains, this area of the body is commonly taped, wrapped or supported in some manner. Following are procedures which can be used to wrap or tape the ankle for protection against injury or support for a weakened or injured ankle. Lace-up supports and semirigid braces are being used more often to support the ankle.

Cloth Ankle Wrap

The cloth ankle wrap gives protection to an uninjured ankle at little expense to the budget by giving mild support to lateral motions at the ankle. The ankle wrap should always be applied over a sock in order to prevent skin irritation due to friction. The wrap is an inelastic cotton webbing, two inches wide and eight to nine feet long. Figure 3-15 illustrates a technique of applying an ankle wrap.

Ankle Wrap

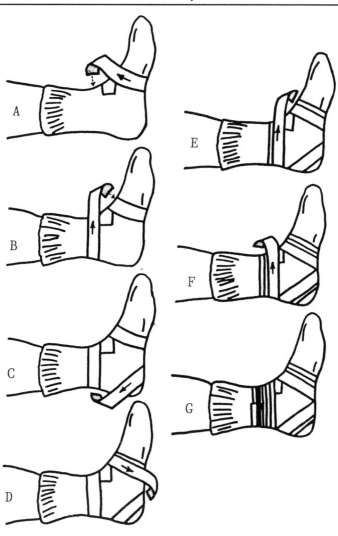

Fig. 3-15

The athlete sits on a table with his or her foot in a functional position, at a 90° angle. Stand facing the sole of the foot and smooth out all wrinkles in the sock. Start the wrap on the instep, continue around the foot (A), and make a figure eight around the ankle joint (B). From the front of the ankle joint, continue the wrap down under the arch, and apply tension as you bring the wrap up and around the back of the heel (C). Tension is applied by pulling the wrap toward the athlete, thus helping to lock the heel.

The wrap continues around the leg to the front of the ankle joint, under the arch again and up around the opposite side of the heel (D). This completes one sequence of the ankle wrap. A second identical series is completed, and with the remaining wrap encircle the leg just above the ankle joint (F). The cloth wrap can be locked by using adhesive tape to encircle the leg (G) or following the same sequence of maneuvers (B-F) with tape. This second technique provides additional support to the ankle wrap.

An athlete can easily be taught to apply his or her own ankle wrap. Instruct them to stand with his or her foot on a bench or chair with the ankle at 90° and wrap the ankle by following the above procedures. Remember to apply tension to the wrap by pulling up as the wrap locks the heel.

Ankle Taping - Regular

The ankle is probably the most frequently taped joint. There are many different taping techniques and procedures used to support the ankle. Following is an ankle taping routine as well as techniques to reinforce this procedure. The basic ankle taping procedure is called a "regular" and can be used for the prevention of ankle injuries as well as to provide support to a weak or injured ankle (Figure 3-16).

The athlete sits on a table with his or her foot in a functional position, which is usually at a 90° angle. Stand facing the sole of the foot. Quite often some form of padding or protection is provided at the sites indicated by the two large arrows (A). These areas are subjected to much stress during activity, and a skin irritation can easily develop. Normally protection is provided by the addition of small pads, some form of lubricant, and/or underwrap encircling this area.

Begin with an anchor around the leg about six inches above the malleoli (#1). Most supporting strips of tape will start and finish on

Ankle Taping - Regular

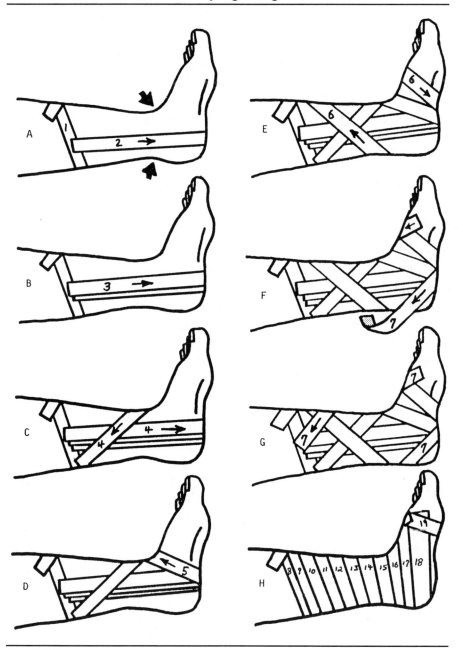

Fig. 3-16

this anchor. Apply two stirrup strips of tape (#2 and #3), starting on the anchor, continuing down and over the malleolus, under the heel, and up along the opposite side of the ankle over the malleolus, and ending on the anchor strip. Since most sprains occur on the outside of the ankle, begin the stirrups on the inside of the leg so the pull is toward the outside.

Strip #4 starts on the inside of the leg, angle the tape forward just slightly and follow the stirrups down under the heel, cross the front of the ankle joint, and continue to the anchor strip. Strip #5 is just the same except it begins on the outside of the leg. Note that these two strips of tape form an "X" just in front of the ankle.

Next come the heel locks. Begin on the top of the foot, continue under the arch, around the heel on the outside, and around the leg to the anchor strip (#6). The inside heel lock (#7) starts on the top of the foot, goes around the heel on the inside, and continues around the leg to the anchor.

Caution: Make sure the tape fits the natural contour of the area and that there are no wrinkles or gaps especially at the areas indicated by the arrows. Tape applied incorrectly can cause small cuts in the skin.

Strips #8 through #18 are lock strips which encircle the ankle and leg from the original anchor strip to the heel. These lock strips should overlap each other approximately one-half. Make certain there are no open areas in the taping procedure as an irritation or blister may develop. A strip of tape around the foot (#19) should lock the loose ends of tape, thus completing the "regular" taping procedure.

Caution: Simply lay strip #19 around the foot, avoiding all pressure along the fifth metatarsal. Undue pressure along this area can become very uncomfortable for the athlete.

Athletic trainers use various methods of reinforcing or adding additional support to a basic ankle taping technique. The amount of support added will depend upon the nature and severity of the injury, the size of the athlete, the activity in which the athlete is involved, and the amount of tape an athlete will tolerate or endure. Remember, to provide support to an area you must limit motion at the involved joints. Providing sufficient support to the ankle may require that you add additional heel locks or more support strips while keeping the tape job comfortable and functional. Here are a couple of methods commonly used to add support to a basic ankle taping technique. Each of these are used in conjunction with a basic ankle tape job and can also be used in combinations.

Outside and Inside Supports

An "outside" or "inside" support is used to provide the ankle further support such as with a recently sprained ankle. The outside support is used to give additional support to the outside or lateral ligaments, while the inside support provides additional support to the deltoid ligament complex. These supports are applied in addition to the regular taping technique and are normally applied just before the lock strips. They can also be applied after the tape job is finished to provide more support. However, they must then be locked down by several more strips of tape encircling the leg.

The outside support is illustrated in Figure 3-17. Note: To make this illustration easier to follow, it is not shown over a tape job as it normally would be. The procedure begins on the bottom of the foot with the roll of tape to the outside (A). The tape is brought around the front of the ankle (B) and forms a figure eight around the leg and foot (C). The tape then continues under the heel and up the outside of the leg in a long stirrup over the lateral malleolus (D). Tension is applied to the tape by pulling the stirrup toward the athlete. This taping technique supports the lateral ligaments.

Outside Support

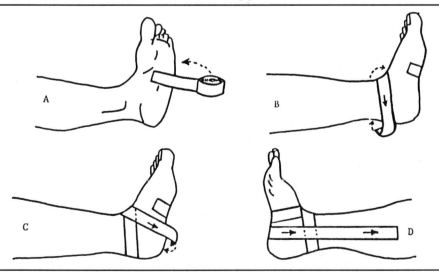

Fig. 3-17

The inside support is identical, except that it starts on the bottom of the foot with the roll of tape to the inside and finishes with a stirrup up the inside of the leg. The type and number of supports used will depend upon the injury and the athlete's preference.

Ankle Figure Eights

Many athletic trainers apply figure eights to provide additional support to an ankle. This maneuver is applied over a basic ankle taping procedure and can be put on before or after the lock strips. The figure eights will provide additional support at the ankle joint and limit plantar flexion. The technique is performed by looping the tape around the foot and leg as indicated in Figure 3-18. Remember to follow the natural contour of the ankle area. Some trainers choose to perform heel locks in conjunction with figure eights. This procedure requires more experience in taping to be able to follow the contours.

Ankle Figure Eights

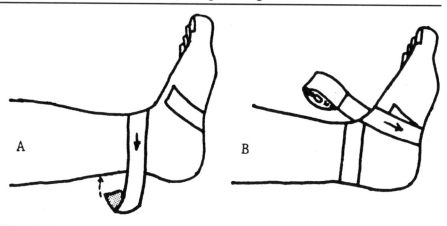

A   B

Fig. 3-18

LEG

The leg is that part of the anatomy from the ankle to the knee. It is composed of the tibia and fibula, which furnishes points of attachment for both thigh and leg muscles and transmits the body weight to the ankle and foot. The muscles of the leg are divided by thick fascial sheaths into four distinct compartments: (1) **anterior**, (2) **lateral**, (3) **deep posterior**, and (4) **superficial posterior**. The calf muscles (gastrocnemius and soleus) are attached to the calcaneus by the largest tendon in the body, the Achilles. The leg is a frequent site for athletic related injuries, especially overuse conditions.

LEG INJURIES

Contusions

The leg is exposed to various types of direct trauma during athletic activity and is therefore subjected to frequent contusions. Contusions occur most often over the shin, where the tibia lies subcutaneously. Bone periosteum is extremely sensitive, and a blow to this area can be very painful and disabling. There is hardly ever a doubt as to the mechanism of injury, that is, a history of direct impact. Contusions to the shin are often associated with abrasions or lacerations resulting from direct trauma. Once the possibility of direct bone injury has been eliminated by the evaluation process, the area should be treated using standard treatment procedures and protected from further trauma.

Contusions can also involve the muscular areas of the leg. A possible complication of a severe contusion to any of the leg muscles is significant swelling within the various compartments. In these closed spaces, swelling is not only uncomfortable but may also lead to a compartment syndrome, which is discussed later. Another possible complication of a direct blow to the leg is damage to the peroneal nerve. This nerve is particularly vulnerable as it passes around the head of the fibula. A severe blow to this area may cause peroneal nerve injury, with pain radiating throughout the distribution of the nerve. Transient tingling and numbness to the lateral surface of the leg or dorsal surface of the foot may remain for a period of time. These symptoms are often temporary and recovery is usually complete.

Strains

Because the leg is the site of origin for the muscles responsible for transmitting power to the foot and ankle, muscle strains are common. These strains result from violent muscular contractions, overstretching or continued overuse. The most common leg strains occur to the calf muscles, usually in the area of the musculotendinous junction or at the insertion of the Achilles tendon into the calcaneus. Strains to the Achilles tendon have a tendency to become chronic and the athlete may develop Achilles tendinitis. Like any other chronic overuse syndrome, Achilles tendinitis requires rest, modification of activity and support during participation.

The Achilles tendon can be supported by the taping procedure illustrated in Figure 3-19. This taping method is designed to shorten action of the tendon and prevent overstretching. The athlete should lie face down with the foot hanging relaxed over the table. An anchor (#1) is applied around the leg about six inches above the malleoli and another (#2) encircles the ball of the foot. Start a support strip of tape (#3) on the anchor around the foot and pull it up over the heel to the anchor around the leg. Elastic tape is often used for this support strip. Take most of the stretch out of the tape as it is applied. Additional strips of tape (#4-#5) are applied the same as strip #3 except that they fan out a little wider at both anchors. When using non-elastic tape for these supports, remember to lay the tape on loose or you may limit too much dorsiflexion. Note: these support strips should be placed directly on the skin so they do not slip.

Achilles Tendon Taping

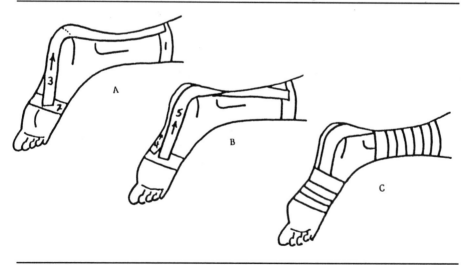

Fig. 3-19

It is very important to lock the support strips down well to prevent slippage and loss of protection. Lock the support strips with several strips of tape encircling the ball of the foot and around the leg (C). The Achilles tendon tape job is often placed under a regular ankle taping procedure which helps lock it in place.

Occasionally the Achilles tendon will rupture. This can result from a single violent contraction or repeated strains. A complete rupture should be readily recognized, as there is often a palpable gap in the tendon and loss of function of the calf muscle. The athlete will also exhibit a positive Thompson test, which is used to evaluate the continuity of the Achilles tendon. This test is accomplished by having the athlete lay prone with his or her feet extended beyond the edge of the table. Squeeze both calves just below their widest circumference and note the reaction of the feet (Figure 3-20). A normal response is that the ankle will plantar flex. If, however, the Achilles tendon is ruptured, the injured side will not respond.

Other muscles of the leg can also become strained during athletic activity. The more common of these are the tibialis anterior and posterior muscles. Symptoms include tenderness at the site of injury and increased pain on active and resistive movements. When these muscles are strained due to continued overuse, they often become inflamed, develop a tendinitis, and are frequently grouped under the heading shin splints.

Thompson Test

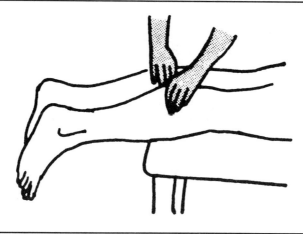

Fig. 3-20

Shin Splints

The term shin splints is unique to the leg. This broad category is a catch all term for chronic painful conditions which occur in the leg. Shin splints most often occur early in a training program or after training has been discontinued for a period of time and then resumed. It appears to be associated with repetitive activity on hard surfaces or forcible excessive use of the leg muscles, especially in running and jumping activities. There is disagreement as to the exact nature and cause of this extremely common condition; however, shin splints are considered to be an overuse syndrome generally limited to the musculotendinous components. Pain associated with shin splints may occur anywhere in the leg and occasionally will become totally disabling. Tenderness is most often found along the medial border of the tibia, which is the origin for the tibialis posterior muscle. There may be any number of causes of shin splints, such as muscle inflexibility, a fallen longitudinal arch, a pronated foot, ill-fitting footwear, training techniques, and playing surfaces. Treatment procedures must emphasize the correction or modification of possible causes. There is no one best treatment for shin splints, and you cannot simply treat the symptoms.

Normally, there are four possible causes for shin splints: (1) muscle strain, (2) stress syndrome, (3) stress fracture, and/or (4) compartment syndrome. Muscle strains were briefly discussed previously. Stress syndromes and stress fractures occur to bone, which is a dynamic tissue, constantly remodeling itself. Excessive stress at a particular point or area can cause the bone to weaken (stress syndrome) or perhaps partially break (stress fracture). It is difficult to define exactly at what point you stop calling the injury a stress syndrome and call it a stress fracture. However, a stress syndrome normally exhibits tenderness over a larger area on the bone while a stress fracture has one tender spot. Both of these conditions indicate overuse and require rest and/or modification of activity.

There are many methods of treating and supporting an athlete for shin splints. Since shin splints are frequently caused by an athlete doing too much too soon in the training program, it is important to attempt to determine what is causing the symptoms and alleviate these problems. The best treatment is to rest the area and modify the training program. Often some type of taping procedure is used to support the painful area. Figure 3-21 illustrates two of the more common taping methods: (A) encircling the leg, with or without a pad, and (B) a spiral technique beginning in the arch area. The tape should cover the painful area as well as a little more area on either side. Occasionally it is also helpful to tape the longitudinal arch as previously illustrated and discussed.

Taping for Shin Splints

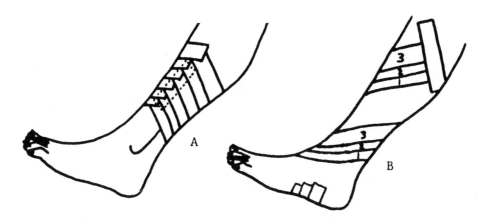

Fig. 3-21

Compartment Syndromes

As previously mentioned, there are four natural compartments in the leg, which contain the muscles, blood vessels, and nerves. The tight binding of fascia that forms these compartments does not allow for significant swelling within their confines. Compartment syndromes can develop whenever there is increased pressure within these tightly confined spaces. This pressure can be caused by swelling due to an inflammatory response resulting from overuse, contusion, or infection. Anything that causes an inflammatory response or uncontrolled swelling may result in increased pressure within one of these compartments. Acute compartment syndromes with severe pain as the result of muscle and nerve ischemia should be readily recognized. It is important to recognize symptoms early and seek medical attention quickly as any delay in treatment may result in permanent neurologic disability.

Another possible cause of compartment syndrome is muscle hypertrophy. As muscles in these tightly confined compartments become bigger as a result of repetitive use or exercise, the relative space decreases, which may give rise to constriction forces. Depending on the cause of the condition there may be sudden or gradual onset of symptoms in the involved leg. There will be swelling accompanied by tenderness and pain in the affected muscle group. In the later stages, numbness, weakness, decreased pulses in the foot, and the inability to use the affected muscle may develop. Any athlete with lower leg symptoms that do not respond to treatment should be reevaluated frequently. Athletes complaining of a constant aching pain that does not completely disappear with rest and becomes more intense with activity should be referred to medical assistance. Compression tests within the involved compartment may be required to recognize the presence of a compartment syndrome.

KNEE

The knee is the largest and considered one of the more complex joints in the body. This hinge joint is the fulcrum of the body's longest lever system. The knee joint is complex because it provides great movement in only one direction (flexion and extension) and restriction in all others. This joint is subjected to tremendous torsional forces and loads during athletic activity and is the site of many athletic injuries and related conditions.

The tibiofemoral joint is the largest in the body and is made up of the articulations between the vertically apposed ends (condyles) of the femur and tibia (Figure 3-22). The bones alone articulate in a precariously unstable way. It is the compensating reinforcement provided by the joint capsule, cartilages, ligaments, and numerous muscle tendons that provides the knee with the security and stability so essential for successful performance in athletic activity. The patellofemoral joint is between the patella and femoral condyles. This gliding type joint is frequently involved in conditions causing anterior knee pain.

Right Knee (anterior view)

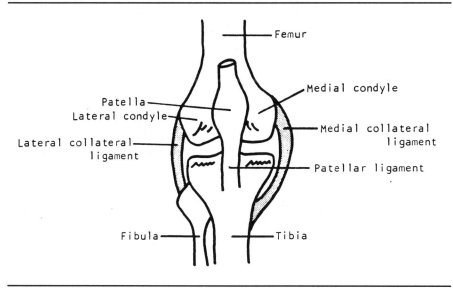

Fig. 3-22

JOINT (SYNOVIAL) CAVITY

The joint cavity of the knee is the largest joint space in the body. The space surrounds the articulating bony condyles and extends three finger-breadths above the patella. The knee joint cavity normally contains 1 to 3 ml of synovial fluid. In addition to providing lubrication for the joint surfaces, synovial fluid provides most of the nutrition for the articular cartilage. The volume can be greatly increased as a result of an athletic injury causing hemorrhaging into the joint cavity or by inflammation of the synovial membrane which increases theproduction of synovial fluid. This increased volume is called **joint effusion**.

COLLATERAL LIGAMENTS

The medial and lateral sides of the knee joint are reinforced by the collateral ligaments (Figure 3-22). These ligaments provide lateral stability, preventing abnormal movement of the knee from side to side. The medial collateral ligament (tibial collateral) is a strong flat band that extends from the medial tubercle of the femur to the medial condyle and shaft of the tibia. This ligament is divided into two layers—superficial and deep. Fibers from the deep layer blend into and fuse with both the joint capsule and medial meniscus. The primary function of the medial collateral ligament is to provide stability against abnormal movements of the knee to the inside. The ligament is tightest on complete extension; however, because it is a flat band, some of its fibers provide support throughout the range of motion.

The medial collateral ligament is the most frequently injured ligament in the knee. The most common cause of injury is a blow to the outside of the knee, which stresses the medial structures as illustrated in Figure 3-23. The medial collateral ligament can also be injured due to rotational stresses.

Blow to Outside of Knee

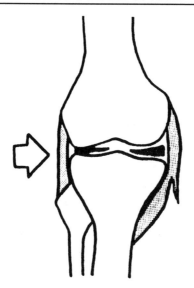

Fig. 3-23

The lateral collateral ligament (fibular collateral) is a rounded, pencil-like cord that extends from the lateral condyle of the femur to the head of the fibula. There is no attachment between the lateral meniscus and the lateral collateral ligament. Unlike its medial counterpart, the lateral collateral ligament is not part of the joint capsule and plays a less significant role in joint stability. It is tight and contributes to stability when the knee is extended, but becomes slack during flexion.

Much of the lateral support of the knee is provided by a structure called the **iliotibial band**. This structure is the distal attachment of the tensor fascia lata muscle, which originates at the iliac crest and posterior aspect of the sacrum. As it passes over the thigh in the region of the greater trochanter it condenses into a broad thick band of fascia called the iliotibial band. As it passes down the lateral aspect of the thigh it attaches indirectly to the distal femur just above the lateral condyle and then crosses the knee and inserts into the upper end of the tibia. The iliotibial band is often considered to be the true lateral collateral ligament and serves as a strong static stabilizer of the lateral side of the knee.

CRUCIATE LIGAMENTS

The cruciate ligaments are relatively short but strong, rounded bands that cross each other, forming an "X" within the joint capsule. They are located between the articular surfaces of the tibial and femoral condyles and are named according to their tibial attachments (Figure 3-24). The role of the cruciate ligaments is complex; however, their primary function is to provide anteroposterior stability. They also function to stabilize the knee from rotational stresses, excessive hyperextension, and abduction and adduction forces. These ligaments are most taut when the knee is in full extension, but some fibers of both cruciates are always tight throughout thefull ROM.

Right Knee (lateral view)

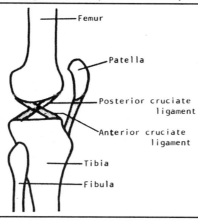

Fig. 3-24

The anterior cruciate ligament attaches to the anterior part of the tibia and then crosses upward and backward to attach on the posterior aspect of the femur. This ligament is primarily responsible for preventing anterior displacement of the tibia on the femur. The ligament is most often injured by a twisting maneuver, forced hyperextension, or lateral blow to the knee.

The posterior cruciate ligament attaches posteriorly to the tibia and extends upward and forward to attach on the anterior femur. This ligament is primarily responsible for preventing posterior displacement of the tibia on the femur. The posterior cruciate appears to be located in the center of the joint and to function as the axis about which the knee moves, both in flexion-extension and rotation. Therefore, it is the fundamental stabilizer of the knee. The posterior is shorter and approximately twice as strong as the anterior cruciate. Therefore, this ligament is not injured as frequently.

MENISCI

The medial and lateral menisci are crescent-shaped pads of fibrocartilage attached to the flat top of the tibia. Because of their concavity, they form a shallow socket for the condyles of the femur. These cartilages enhance the total stability of the knee, assist in the control of normal knee motion, and provide shock absorption against compression forces between the tibia and femur. The peripheral border of each meniscus is thick, convex, and attached to the inside capsule of the joint. The opposite border tapers to a thin, free edge.

The medial meniscus is a larger and more oval or "C"-shaped cartilage located on the inside of the knee (Figure 3-25). This cartilage is also more firmly fixed to the tibia and capsule which results in it being injured more frequently. Because of its attachment to the medial collateral ligament, the medial meniscus may also be injured in conjunction with a sprain of this ligament. The lateral meniscus is a smaller and more round or "O"-shaped cartilage on the outside of the knee. It is not as firmly attached and has greater freedom of movement. Therefore the lateral meniscus is not injured as often as the medial meniscus.

Menisci of Knee

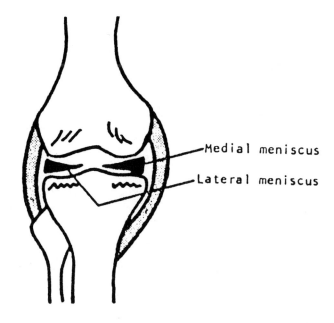

Medial meniscus

Lateral meniscus

Fig. 3-25

The menisci are frequently injured or torn as they become trapped, pinched, or crushed between the femoral condyles and the tibial plateaus. The damage sustained can be quite varied, ranging from a very small tear (Figure 3-26, A & B) to a large longitudinal tear resulting in a displaced segment of the cartilage. This type of tear is generally referred to as a **bucket handle tear** (C). Tears around the periphery of the meniscus or to the ligamentous attachments may heal because of the blood supply to this area. Tears involving the avascular body of the meniscus will not heal and usually result in persistent symptoms requiring surgical intervention. When a cartilage is injured, the torn edges harden and a clicking in the knee may develop. Large torn fragments or loose pieces of cartilage may also cause the knee to "lock" causing the knee to have a reduced range of motion. The detached or dislocated cartilage must be removed or reduced to allow the athlete to move his or her knee through a normal range of motion.

Meniscal Injuries

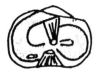   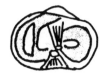

A - Posterior rim tear   B - Transverse tear   C - Longitudinal tear

Fig. 3-26

Figure 3-27 illustrates the arrangement of the anatomical structures discussed so far. Note the relationships of each. A discussion of the common assessment procedures used to evaluate these structures will be presented before continuing with additional injuries to the knee.

Right Knee (superior view)

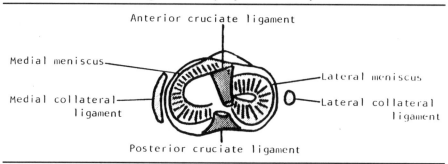

Anterior cruciate ligament

Medial meniscus

Lateral meniscus

Medial collateral ligament

Lateral collateral ligament

Posterior cruciate ligament

Fig. 3-27

COMMON KNEE EVALUATION PROCEDURES

Evaluation of a knee injury should follow the standard procedures of history, observation, and physical examination. While there are many stress procedures used in evaluating knee injuries, this manual will only discuss and illustrate the more common techniques used. After completing the history and inspection of the knee, localize any pain and swelling. To locate pain, gently palpate various areas about the knees to elicit tenderness. Remember, tenderness is normally present at the site of an injury. Evaluate any swelling by gently feeling for fluid. Swelling may be within the joint capsule (effusion) or diffused outside the capsule. Swelling inside the knee joint usually indicates injury to the capsule or structures within. It is important to note the time it takes for effusion to accumulate. Effusion present within a couple of hours following an injury generally indicates that the swelling is due to blood from hemorrhage into the joint cavity. This usually indicates a significant injury such as to the cruciates or cartilages. Effusion that occurs over 12-24 hours is generally excess synovial fluid resulting from the capsule being irritated or inflamed, such as with a collateral ligament injury. An athlete with a joint effusion will frequently hold the injured knee in 30° to 45° of flexion, the point at which the volume of the joint cavity is the greatest, resulting in the injured knee being less painful.

Evaluating for Joint Effusion

To evaluate for joint effusion, begin by placing one hand 3-4 inches above the patella on the thigh and the fingers and thumb of the other hand on the joint line. Run your hand down the thigh, stopping just above the kneecap, to "milk" the upper portion of the joint cavity (Figure 3-28). Then using your fingers, feel for fluid on each side of the knee at the joint line. If there is excess fluid in the joint capsule, you will feel a **fluid wave** on one side of the joint as you push on the opposite side.

Feeling for Joint Effusion

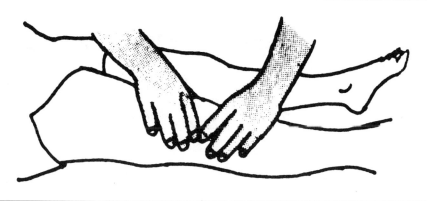

Fig. 3-28

Evaluating Collateral Ligaments

To evaluate those structures that support the inside of the knee, use the **abduction stress test**. This is performed with the athlete laying down with both legs supported by a table or the ground to assist with relaxation and to avoid muscle contraction. To perform the abduction stress test place one hand on the lateral side of the knee and the other hand above the ankle on the medial side (Figure 3-29). Then gently apply lateral force to the ankle and medial stress against the knee in an attempt to abduct the leg and open the knee joint on the inside. Repeat the test, gradually increasing the stress to localize the pain and detect any abnormal looseness in the joint. Look for any separation or laxity at the medial joint line. The abduction stress test should be done first with the knee in complete extension and then again in about 30° of flexion. Remember, the athlete must have the thigh and leg muscles relaxed for you to obtain an accurate evaluation.

To test those structures on the lateral side of the knee, an **adduction stress test** is performed. Reverse the hand position so one hand is on the inside of the knee and the other above the ankle. Medial force is then applied against the ankle and lateral stress against the knee.

Perform these same procedures on the uninjured knee and compare the results. If any abnormal instability is recognized, it probably indicates a torn or partially torn collateral ligament and the athlete should be referred to a physician. Increased tenderness along the ligament without any noticeable abnormal motion, probably indicates the ligament is only stretched.

Abduction Stress Test

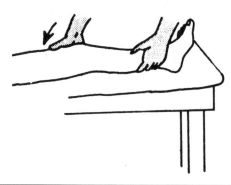

Fig. 3-29

Evaluating Cruciate Ligaments

Evaluating cruciate ligaments normally involves the **drawer test**. This test is performed with the athlete in a comfortable relaxed supine (on back) position. The hip is flexed approximately 45° and the knee is flexed to 90° with the foot resting flat on the table (Figure 3-30). The foot should be in a neutral position, facing straight ahead. Sit on the athlete's foot to stabilize it, cup your hands around the upper tibia and place your thumbs along the medial and lateral joint lines. Palpate the hamstring tendons with your fingers to make sure the muscles are relaxed. Gently pull the tibia forward to perform an anterior drawer test. This test puts stress on the anterior cruciate ligament. If the tibia slides forward, the anterior cruciate ligament has been damaged. Next push the tibia backward to perform the posterior drawer test to evaluate the posterior cruciate ligament. Again compare the results with those from the uninjured knee. If you detect any abnormal motion the athlete should be referred to a physician.

Another test used to evaluate cruciate instability is **Lachman's test**, which may be more reliable than the drawer test. It is particularly useful when muscle relaxation is a problem, because the hamstrings and the iliotibial band have little effect on the outcome. When the knee is flexed 90°, as with the drawer test, the hamstrings directly oppose forward movement of the tibia. If the athlete contracts the hamstrings, or if the muscles are in spasm, there may not be any abnormal movement even though an instability exists.

Drawer Test for Knee

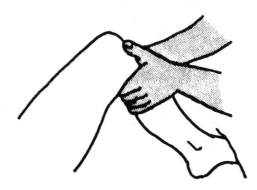

Fig. 3-30

Lachman's test is performed with the athlete supine on the table and the knee flexed 10° to 15°. The femur is stabilized with one hand while the other grasps the upper tibia with the thumb along the joint line, as shown in Figure 3-31. When an athlete's leg is too large or the evaluator's hands too small to grasp the tibia in one hand, the tibia can be held between the arm and the chest of the evaluator. Apply force to the tibia in an attempt to lift it forward and push it backwards or posteriorly. Note any abnormal movement or instability.

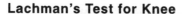

Lachman's Test for Knee

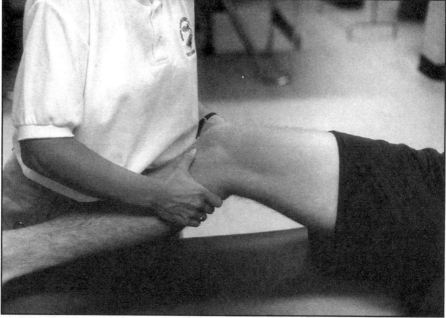

Fig. 3-31

Evaluating Menisci

Determining if an acute knee injury has resulted in a torn cartilage is often difficult, especially if there is also damage to a ligament. Point tenderness along the joint line, especially in the absence of a positive abduction or adduction stress test, may indicate an injury to the meniscus. All tests evaluating meniscal tears are founded on the same mechanical basis, that is, attempting to trap or pinch the injured meniscus between the articular surfaces of the femur and tibia by performing various rotational maneuvers. A torn meniscus may cause pain or a clicking or snapping sensation during these procedures.

Figure 3-32 illustrates the **McMurray test**. This test is performed with the athlete lying supine and the hip and knee flexed maximally. Hold the athlete's heel in one hand and feel the joint line with the thumb and index finger of the other hand. Passively internally and externally rotate the tibia with the hand on the heel while gently forcing the knee medially and laterally to bring the femur into closer approximation with the tibia and cartilages. Passively extend the knee while performing these maneuvers. Feel and listen for any clicking or snapping which may indicate an injury to the meniscus.

McMurray Test

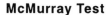

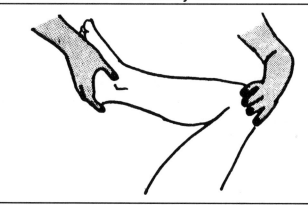

Fig. 3-32

OTHER KNEE INJURIES

There are many other athletic related injuries or conditions that can occur to the knee or surrounding structures. Following is a brief discussion of the more common knee conditions.

Prepatellar Bursitis

The prepatellar bursa lies between the front of the patella and the skin. This is the largest and most commonly injured bursa in the knee. Prepatellar bursitis is a common problem in athletes who suffer repeated trauma to the front of the knee such as falling on the knee or getting hit on the patella. The injured bursa reacts by producing additional bursal fluid resulting in a large amount of fluid accumulating between the kneecap and skin. This condition is often called "water on the knee" and historically has been called "carpet layer's" or "housemaid's" knee. It may not be too painful and often times an athlete will continue activity. Occasionally, the bursa will have to be drained.

Patellar Tendinitis

Patellar tendinitis (**jumper's knee**) is an overuse condition found in many athletes involved in repetitive jumping activities, such as basketball players or high jumpers. It is an inflammatory response to repeated stress or irritation of the patellar tendon at its insertion. This tendinitis is normally characterized by pain localized at the lower (distal) end of the patella. The athlete will complain of pain during activity, especially with excessive quadriceps action. To evaluate for patellar tendinitis apply pressure to the upper edge of the kneecap which causes the lower edge to "wing". Then palpate the insertion of the tendon (Figure 3-33). An athlete with patellar tendinitis will exhibit point tenderness when you palpate this area.

Palpating for Patellar Tendinitis

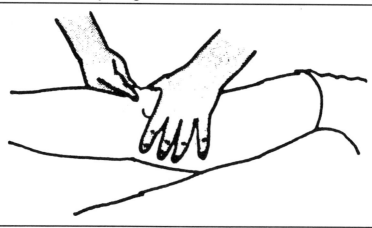

Fig. 3-33

Osgood-Schlatter Syndrome

Osgood-Schlatter's Syndrome is a condition involving the tibial tuberosity of adolescents. It occurs in young athletes where the attachment of the growth plate (epiphysis) of the tibial tuberosity to the shaft of the tibia is the weakest link in the extensor mechanism. Repeated stresses on the patellar tendon causes a minor avulsion of the tibial tuberosity, resulting in an inflammatory reaction. The young athlete will have pain on active use of the quadriceps. On evaluation the athlete will have point tenderness on the tibial tuberosity and pain on resistance to quadriceps action. This condition is usually self-limiting and the athlete will grow out of it eventually. However, an enlarged tibial tuberosity often remains. Normally, a conservative treatment plan consisting of modifying or restricting painful activities, flexibility exercises, and anti-inflammatory care will allow an athlete to continue athletic activity.

Patellar Subluxation

The kneecap may fully dislocate or, more commonly partially dislocate (sublux) during athletic activity. Patellar subluxations almost always move to the outside (lateral) as the patella slides over the lateral femoral condyle. Recurrent subluxations are often associated with either congenital or developmental deficiencies in the quadriceps mechanism or bony configuration. Women are more prone to this condition because of their wider bony pelvis structure and angulated femurs. Symptoms produced by recurrent subluxations are similar to other internal derangements of the knee. The athlete may describe the knee as "giving way," popping or catching. Tenderness is located along the edges of the kneecap and the athlete will exhibit a positive **apprehension test**. This is accomplished by pushing the kneecap outward, attempting to dislocate it laterally. If the patella is prone to subluxating, the athlete will become very apprehensive about this maneuver and resist any attempt to move the kneecap (Figure 3-34).

Apprehension Test

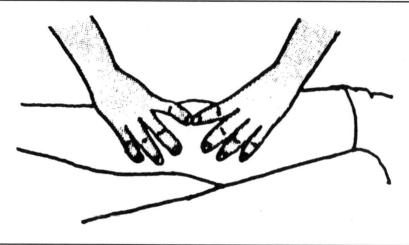

Fig. 3-34

Chondromalacia Patellae

Chondromalacia patellae is a degeneration process that results in a softening of the articular surface of the patella. This condition is normally caused by an irritation of the patellar groove, with subsequent changes occurring in the cartilage on the underside of the kneecap. Many factors can contribute to chondromalacia. The symptoms usually have a gradual onset and progress slowly. The athlete will complain of pain beneath the kneecap, especially during activities requiring flexion of the knee. The athlete may also express a grating or grinding sensation, the knee buckling, an aching pain after vigorous activity, or pain after sitting for a prolonged time. On examination, there is usually tenderness along the edges of the patella, discomfort on compressing the kneecap into the femoral groove, and pain on contraction of the quadriceps against patellar pressure. The athlete may also exhibit swelling, crepitus, and a positive apprehension test.

Iliotibial Band Friction Syndrome

Iliotibial band friction syndrome is a condition frequently seen in runners. This is an inflammatory process or bursitis that develops deep to the iliotibial band as it crosses over the lateral femoral condyle during repetitive activity, such as running. The athlete suffering from this condition complains of pain or tenderness over the lateral femoral condyle.

Peroneal Nerve Contusion

The peroneal nerve passes just below the head of the fibula, where it lies subcutaneously. A direct blow to this area can result in a contusion and injure the nerve, which is caught between the underlying bone and the force. The athlete may exhibit a localized pain from the contusion and a radiating pain to the anterior lateral leg musculature and dorsum of the foot. Numbness and tingling in the distribution of the nerve is also present. Normally the symptoms last only a few seconds or minutes, but in severe cases the hypesthesia and weakness of the peroneals and dorsiflexors persists. The athlete may even develop a foot drop. Usually the contusion of the nerve is minor and symptoms subside within a day or two after the injury.

Epiphyseal injuries

You should be suspicious with any skeletally immature athlete with acute knee trauma for the possibility of an epiphyseal injury. For example, the medial collateral ligament (MCL) attaches on the epiphyseal portion of the femur and the metaphyseal portion of the tibia. This anatomically protects the proximal tibial epiphysis from stress while exposing the distal femoral epiphysis to external forces. An injury mechanism that would cause an MCL sprain in an adult may disrupt the distal femoral epiphyseal plate. It may be difficult to distinguish a ligamentous instability from an epiphyseal fracture. The tenderness should be predominantly over the growth plate. It is a good practice to refer any young athlete with instability or an acute bloody swelling of the knee.

KNEE SUPPORT

The incidence of knee injuries is high, probably second in number to ankle injuries. Because of this high incidence and the wide variety of conditions that occur, many protective and supportive devices have been devised and are utilized for the knee.

Preventative knee braces (Figure 3-35) are the newest devices that are gaining rapid popularity. There are currently many varieties on the market. The more popular braces consist of two rigid halves that are hinged as they cross the outside of the knee. These braces are secured around the thigh and calf and are designed to protect against a lateral blow which is the most common mechanism of knee injury. These have proven to be very beneficial in protecting the knee against injury.

Another very popular support is the knee sleeve (Figure 3-36). These are made of various thicknesses of neoprene rubber which is covered by nylon. These sleeves completely encase the knee area and provide pressure around the knee as well as retain heat. There are also many varieties of knee sleeves. For example, some have felt buttresses sewn into them to assist with tracking of the patella or providing additional pressure over a certain area.

There are also functional braces (Figure 3-37) designed to protect an injured knee or one that has been repaired surgically. These devices are usually expensive and are form fit for each individual athlete. They provide support from lateral forces aswell as rotary stresses.

Preventative Knee Brace	Knee Sleeve	Functional Brace

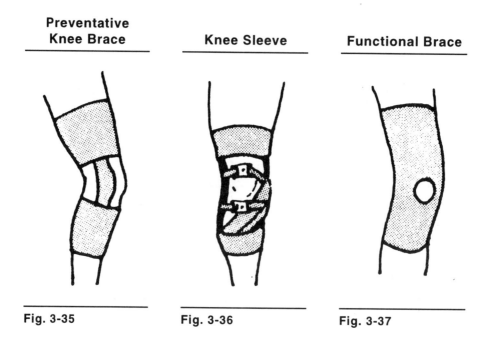

Fig. 3-35　　　　　Fig. 3-36　　　　　Fig. 3-37

TAPING the KNEE

Tape is still widely used to provide support for an injured knee. Some disadvantages of tape are skin irritations, expense, the time it takes to apply and the lack of support afforded to various knee conditions. Therefore, knee sleeves and braces are being utilized more and more. However, taping the knee remains a valuable method of providing support to an injured knee depending upon the type and amount of damage sustained.

Collateral Support

An "X" method of taping is employed to provide support for a mild to moderate collateral ligament injury. Often times elastic tape is used for this basic knee taping procedure because of its ease in application, conforming to leg motion, and strength when compared to regular adhesive tape. If additional support is required, regular adhesive tape can be incorporated over the elastic tape.

Figure 3-38 illustrates the basic "X" taping procedure for medial support. The athlete stands with the affected knee flexed approximately 30°. Strip #1 begins on the outside of the leg, crosses the inside of the knee joint, and finishes on the inside of the thigh. The elastic

Basic X

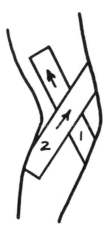

Fig. 3-38

tape should be stretched tightly. Strip #2 starts on the inside of the leg, crosses the knee joint, and ends on the outside of the thigh. These two strips of tape form an "X" at the joint line on the medial side of the knee joint. This may be all the support needed, at which time the elastic tape is locked in place, which is discussed later.

Often a double "X" taping procedure is used. This consists of putting an "X" on both the medial and lateral sides of the knee joint (Figure 3-39). Strips #3 and #4 r epresent the "X" on the lateral side.

If additional support is needed on either the medial or lateral aspect of the knee, additional strips of elastic tape can be applied as described above. Another method of providing additional support is to apply regular adhesive tape over the elastic tape. During activity, regular adhesive tape is easily torn where it crosses the knee joint if it is not twisted or folded. Figure 3-40 illustrates the application of twisted tape to reinforce the basic knee taping. The tape is twisted a couple of times to form a small cord and applied with tension. Where these twists cross each other (X) should coincide with the center of motion (axis) of the knee or movement will be restricted. The number of twists applied will be determined by the athlete's tolerance. The athlete should bear weight on the knee, moving it from side to side, and inform you when the support is sufficient. Remember, the more tape you put on, the more support you give the athlete, but the more motion you take away.

Double X   **Twisted Tape**

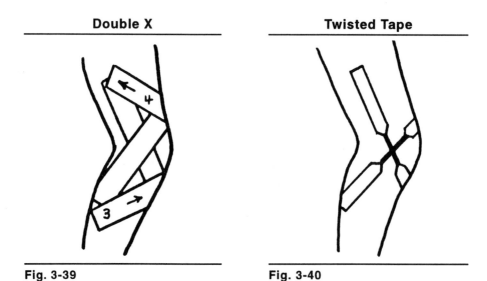

Fig. 3-39   **Fig. 3-40**

If elastic tape is too expensive, or not available, the basic knee taping procedure employing regular adhesive tape should be followed. A basketweave taping method using regular adhesive tape is illustrated in Figure 3-41. The regular tape must be twisted or folded where it crosses the center of motion of the joint or it will probably tear during activity. Again, tape is applied until the athlete states the support is sufficient.

Caution: Never apply twisted tape directly over the skin as it will cause irritation during activity. Make certain there is at least one layer of flat tape between the skin and twisted tape.

Locking the basic knee taping procedure in place can be accomplished by various methods. Figure 3-42 illustrates using elastic tape to encircle the leg and thigh and lock all loose ends. The kneecap and back of the knee should be left open. The end of the elastic tape must be locked with regular adhesive tape because it does not adhere to itself adequately.

Figure 3-43 illustrates using regular adhesive tape to lock the support strips in position. These lock strips do not encircle the leg completely as they may become constrictive when the athlete is engaged in activity. Leave a small gap between the ends of the lock strips (A). An elastic bandage should be applied over the taping procedure to secure all the loose ends (B).

Basketweave for Knee	Locking with Elastic Tape	Locking with Regular Tape

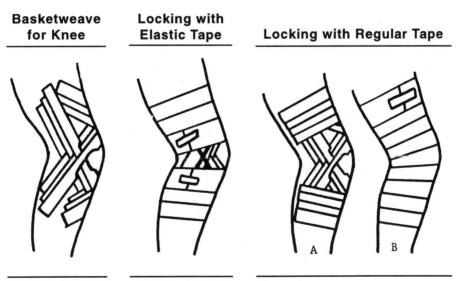

Fig. 3-41	Fig. 3-42	Fig. 3-43

Hyperextension Support

Figure 3-44 illustrates a taping procedure designed to prevent the knee from being hyperextended. This method is used to help protect pulled hamstring tendons, stretched cruciate ligaments, and other injuries that may cause pain upon complete extension of the knee joint. This procedure can also be used in conjunction with the collateral ligament taping method.

Taping for Hyperextension of the Knee

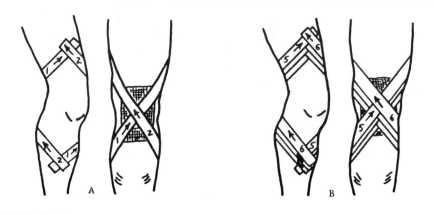

Fig. 3-44

Have the athlete stand on a table with the injured knee flexed about 30°. A gauze pad should be placed behind the knee joint to protect the area from irritation caused by the tape.

Strip #1 begins about six to eight inches directly below the patella, continues up and around the back of the knee, and ends about six to eight inches directly above the patella. Strip #2 begins and ends at the same points as #1, but it continues around the knee in the opposite direction. These two strips of tape should form an "X" behind the knee joint (A). Additional strips of tape are applied, similar to the first two, depending upon the severity of the injury and the size of the athlete (B).

The hyperextension taping procedure is locked similarly to the collateral taping method using either elastic or regular adhesive tape.

THIGH

The femur, the long single bone of the thigh, is surrounded by thick musculature. The major muscles of the thigh are the quadriceps in front and the hamstrings in back. These muscles are subjected to extreme stresses during most athletic activity and are vulnerable to impact forces, especially during contact sports. As a result, the thigh is an area of the body commonly injured during athletics.

Thigh Contusions

Contusions to the anterior thigh, or quadriceps, occur frequently due to a direct blow to this area. This injury is frequently called a **"charley horse"**. Symptoms can range from mild tenderness with little restriction of motion to marked pain, swelling, and restricted motion or function. A potentially problem with thigh contusions is delayed or silent bleedingwithin the injured muscle that may continue for varying periods of time. In these cases the full extent of the injury may not be recognized for 12 to 24 hours. Frequently the athlete will continue activity during this time, and only after re-evaluation the following day will the severity of the injury be recognized. The signs and symptoms associated with thick-muscle injuries are often less localized than in other more subcutaneous areas of the body.

A complication to be aware of when handling thigh contusions is **myositis ossificans**. This is the formation of bone within or around a muscle, commonly called a calcium deposit. Myositis ossificans results when part of the hematoma fails to be absorbed by the body and is replaced with bone. This can occur anywhere in the body but more frequently involves the quadriceps. The complication is more likely to occur after a chronic irritation, such as continued use of the injured quadriceps or repeated contusions. This condition should be suspected if the hematoma fails to resolve and pain, swelling, and loss of motion persist for 2-3 weeks.

Thigh contusions need to be protected when the athlete returns to activity. This is usually in the form of a thigh pad or a large, donut-shaped vinyl foam rubber pad with a hard covering to prevent the bruised area from receiving further blows. These protective pads can be held in place with an elastic wrap encircling the area.

Thigh Strains

Muscle strains are another common thigh injury. The type of sudden violent contractions or stretching of muscles associated with running and jumping activities frequently results in strains. Conditions which may contribute to muscle strains are lack of flexibility, fatigue, inadequate warm-up, muscle weaknesses, deficiency in the reciprocal action of opposing muscles, or imbalance between quadriceps and hamstring strength. The severity of thigh strains may range from muscle cramps to complete tears, or ruptures. The hamstring muscles are strained more frequently than the quadriceps. This type of injury tends to recur and frequently becomes a chronic problem. The signs and symptoms associated with thigh strains are pain, tenderness, muscle spasm, and loss of function, motion and/or strength. Usually these signs and symptoms are intensified by active and resistive motions.

A strained hamstring is usually supported by a snugly applied elastic wrap or sleeve. Often a foam rubber pad is placed over the pulled area as indicated in Figure 3-45. This provides compression and further support for this area.

Wrapping for a Pulled Hamstring

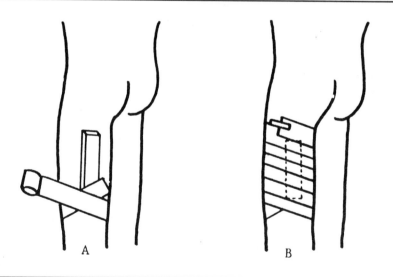

A   B

Fig. 3-45

HIP

The hip area or pelvic girdle consists of the two coxal bones, commonly called the pelvic, innominate, or hip bones. Each of these bones consists of three components or bones which become fused together, the ilium, ischium and pubis (Figure 3-46). The coxal bones are united to each other anteriorly at the pubic symphysis and posteriorly to the sacrum. Together they form the pelvic girdle which provides a strong and stable support for the lower extremities.

Right Hip (anterior view)

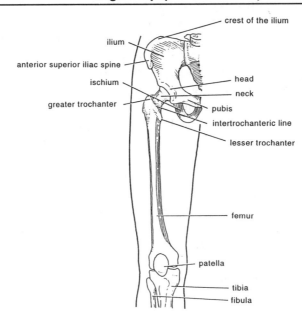

crest of the ilium
ilium
anterior superior iliac spine
ischium
greater trochanter
head
neck
pubis
intertrochanteric line
lesser trochanter
femur
patella
tibia
fibula

Fig. 3-46

The hip joint is made up of the head of the femur and the acetabulum, which is the cup-shaped socket of the innominate or coxal bone. The articular capsule that encloses the hip joint is quite dense and very strong. It is reinforced by three ligaments: (1) iliofemoral (considered the strongest ligament in the body), (2) pubofemoral, and (3) ischiofemoral. These three ligaments come off the three fused bones that form the pelvis, and spiral around the neck of the femur. They become taut on full extension.

The hip is one of the strongest and most stable joints in the body. Athletic injuries to this joint are relatively uncommon.

Hip Contusions

The most common contusion to the hip occurs to the iliac crest, commonly called a **hip pointer**. This crest is the most subcutaneous area of the hip and is especially susceptible to direct blows during contact sports. A hip pointer can involve the hip muscles that originate along its outer border or the abdominals that attach along the upper and inner border. A hip pointer is a painful and handicapping injury since any movement increases the pain.

Contusions to the crest of the ilium need to be protected and supported when the athlete returns to activity. This area is usually protected with the use of a hard shelled pad to disperse any blows to the area. The area can also be supported by the use of tape in an attempt to decrease some of the painful motion.

Figure 3-47 illustrates a method of taping for support of a hip pointer. Alternating strips of tape are pulled up over the crest of the ilium (A & B). These strips should run from the midline in front of the body to the midline in back. Begin below the site of injury and crisscross the tape up and over the injured area. Next, horizontal strips should be applied over the crossing tape (C). Again go from midline to midline. Finish the taping procedure by encircling the waist with an elastic wrap to secure the tape (D).

Taping for a Hip Pointer

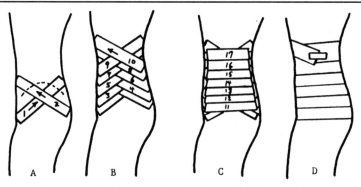

A   B   C   D

Fig. 3-47

Hip Strains

Of the muscles about the hip, those which compose the groin are injured most frequently during athletic activity. The groin is the body area lying between the thigh and abdomen and the muscle in this region consist of the hip adductors and flexors. Muscle strains involving these muscles are common in all athletic activities that involve running, especially those characterized by sudden bursts of speed and cutting maneuvers. Groin strains are commonly caused by a violent muscle contraction or overstretching. The athlete may report feeling a sudden twinge or stretching sensation in the groin. In other instances, initial symptoms may be mild and the athlete may not notice or report the injury until after the activity is completed.

The signs and symptoms of a groin strain are similar to those of other muscle strains. Supporting an athlete when returning to activity is often accomplished with the use of the flexed hip spica wrap which was illustrated in Figure 1-14. This is a good method of supporting the groin musculature.

Trochanteric Bursitis

The bony greater trochanter is covered only by the trochanteric bursa and tensor fascia latae muscle. The function of the bursa is to lessen friction as the tensor fascia latae slides over the trochanter during movement. A direct blow to the trochanter may result in a contusion of the muscle or lead to **trochanteric bursitis**. Friction within the bursa caused by the tensor fascia latae muscle constantly gliding over the trochanter can also result in bursitis. Palpating the greater trochanter will cause pain with both a contusion and trochanteric bursitis. However, if the bursa is inflamed, movements forcing the tensor fascia latae muscle over the trochanter will cause pain. Chronic trochanteric bursitis with thickening of the bursal walls can cause a condition known as a **snapping hip**. As the tensor fascia latae slides back and forth over the trochanteric bursa, an audible and palpable snap will occur. This condition is more common in women because they have a wider pelvis and a more prominent trochanter.

INJURIES TO THE AXIAL REGION

Athletic related injuries to the axial region are not nearly as common as to the extremities. However, injuries involving this region are extremely important because this area contains the vital organs of the circulatory, respiratory, nervous, and digestive systems of the body. The axial division of the body includes the torso (abdominal and thoracic subdivisions), spine and head. Injuries involving these areas can be life threatening or cause permanent damage.

TORSO

The torso of the body is composed of two major areas: (1) the **abdomen**, and (2) the **thorax** (chest). The boundary between these two is the diaphragm, and each area forms a major body cavity containing life sustaining organs. Athletic injuries can occur to either the walls of these cavities or their visceral contents. Superficial injuries involving the cavity walls are much more common during athletic activity and are generally not serious. Fortunately, athletic injuries to the internal contents of either of these cavities are not common. However, serious and potentially life threatening injuries can occur. You must be alert for the possibilities of serious internal injuries resulting from athletic activity.

ABDOMEN

The abdomen is that portion of the body torso bounded above by the diaphragm and below by the upper pelvis. The abdominal cavity is continuous with the pelvic cavity and its wall merges with the wall of the pelvis below and the thorax above. The abdominal area is vulnerable to injury during most activities, especially contact sports. The muscular abdominal wall is the most commonly involved area. Occasionally the underlying visceral contents may be involved, which can be serious.

Abdominal Contusions

Contusions are common to the abdominal muscles as this area can be easily subjected to direct blows during many types of athletic activity. Because of the resiliency of the abdominal wall, muscle contusions are generally not serious. No rigid background exists on which an external blow can impact. The greatest danger of impact-type trauma to the abdominal wall is injury to the contents within the cavity.

Abdominal Strains

Strains of the abdominal muscles are usually the result of a sudden violent contraction, overstretching, or continued overuse. Signs and symptoms include localized tenderness, muscle spasm, and rigidity. The pain will be increased or aggravated by active muscular contraction or passive stretching. For this reason, strains of the abdominal muscles tend to be disabling because these muscles are important when performing most athletic activities. Abdominal strains do not usually involve tearing of the muscle fibers and recovery is generally rapid.

Side Ache

Another common condition involving the abdominal wall is a side ache or "stitch in the side." The sharp pain and muscle spasms associated with this condition usually occur along the lower rib cage or in the upper abdominal muscles. Side aches are often associated with running activities and are usually short lived. The pain is usually relieved after cessation of the activity and also responds well to stretching the involved side. There are several possible causes of side aches but it is generally believed that most are caused by a spasm of the diaphragm. Contributing factors may be level of condition, current training program, eating habits, or elimination routines.

Wind Knocked Out

Another common occurrence in the abdominal region is a blow to the **solar (celiac) plexus** resulting in having the "wind knocked out." The solar plexus is a network of nerves lying deep in the upper middle region of the abdomen. A blow to this area can cause a transitory paralysis of the diaphragm. Although an athlete may become very anxious, this injury is usually of very short duration, and no treatment is necessary because the condition responds to a few minutes of rest and reassurance.

Hernia

The protrusion of abdominal viscera through the abdominal wall is called a hernia. This condition, while generally not caused by an athletic injury, can be aggravated by athletic activity, such as weight training or strenuous activity. The areas of the abdominal wall most susceptible to hernias are the inguinal and femoral canals. The inguinal canal is the point at which the spermatic cord containing blood vessels, nerves, and the vas deferens of the male reproductive system leaves the abdominal cavity and enters the scrotum. In the female, the round ligament of the uterus passes through the canal and terminates in the labia majora. The femoral canal is the point at which the femoral blood vessels and nerve pass from the abdominal cavity into the lower extremity. These two openings are protected by muscular control, much like the shutter of a camera. They may be congenitally weak or weakened by increased intra-abdominal pressure, resulting in abdominal viscera being forced through these canals. Symptoms associated with a hernia include pain and prolonged discomfort as well as a feeling of weakness or pulling in the groin. A protrusion may be felt, which will increase on coughing and decrease when the athlete reclines. Suspected hernias should be referred to a physician.

Genitalia Injuries

Athletic injuries to the genitalia, and especially to the internal reproductive organs, are extremely uncommon. The female reproductive structures being almost entirely internal and well protected by the bony pelvis and abdominal musculature, are seldom injured. A more common injury occurs to the external genitalia of the male athlete. The testes are fairly vulnerable to injury during many types of athletic activity. These injuries usually occur as the result of a direct blow to the scrotum. The resulting contusion can range from very mild to an extremely painful, nauseating, and disabling injury for the athlete. In most cases, pain is short lived. The athlete may complain of a drawing or pulling sensation as the muscles supporting the testes go into spasm.

Following a blow to the scrotum, the athlete must be put at ease and testicular spasm reduced. One method of reducing testicular spasm is to instruct or assist the athlete in bringing both knees up toward his chest. This assists in relaxing the muscle spasms and reducing discomfort. Another procedure that helps reduce testicular spasm is the **Valsalva maneuver**. This is accomplished when the athlete forcibly exhales against a closed glottis, thereby building up intra-abdominal pressure. Examine for or have the athlete check for normal positioning and appearance of the testes following a blow to the scrotum. It is possible that torsion of the spermatic cord can occur by a testicle revolving in the scrotum as a result of trauma. If this condition has occurred, the scrotum may appear to be a cluster of swollen veins, and the athlete may experience a dull pain combined with a heavy, dragging sensation in the scrotal region. An athlete with these signs and symptoms should receive immediate medical attention. Usually the signs and symptoms associated with most scrotal injuries subside in a few minutes and require no further evaluation. If the trauma results in residual pain and swelling, the athlete should use an athletic supporter for scrotal support during the recovery phase. Continue to monitor this athlete and if symptoms persist or become worse, the athlete should be referred to medical assistance for further evaluation and treatment.

Intra-abdominal Injuries

Athletic injuries involving the contents of the abdominal cavity occur infrequently. However, as mentioned previously, these injuries can become life threatening. These injuries are usually associated with contact or collision sports and occur as the result of some type of direct trauma to the abdomen or lower back. The structures most often associated with serious intra-abdominal injuries are the solid organs such as the kidneys, spleen, and liver; all organs rich in blood supply. Occasionally the hollow organs, mesentery, peritoneum, or female reproductive organs are involved in an athletic injury. Intra-abdominal injuries or conditions can develop quickly or insidiously over a period of time; therefore, you must be alert to signs and symptoms that may indicate possible intra-abdominal involvement.

An athlete who has sustained an injury to the abdomen and exhibits any of the following signs and symptoms should be referred to medical assistance.

1. Pain or discomfort increasing in the abdomen
2. Rigidity and spasm of abdominal muscles
3. Blood in the urine or stool
4. Referred pain and rebound tenderness
5. Increased nausea
6. Vomiting
7. Painful urination
8. Signs of shock

THORAX

The chest or thoracic cavity is surrounded by a bony cage formed by the sternum anteriorly, the ribs laterally and the thoracic vertebrae posteriorly. Within this bony cage are the lungs, heart, and great vessels. These structures are well protected and not often involved in athletic injuries.

Chest Wall

The majority of athletic injuries to the thorax are superficial, involving the chest wall or rib age. Most result from a direct blow to the area. Contusions or bruises are the most frequent injuries to the chest wall. They may involve the skin, subcutaneous tissues, muscles, or periosteum of the ribs or sternum. On examination, contusions to the chest wall reveal an area of localized tenderness and possibly swelling. In most instances this type of injury does not cause pain during breathing or restrict motion of the rib cage unless very deep respirations are taken.

Another possible injury is a rib fracture. These are usually caused by a direct blow but can also result from a forceful compression of the rib cage. Ribs 4 through 9 are most likely to be fractured, since the first three ribs are protected by the shoulder girdle. The lower ribs (10 through 12) also have a greater freedom of movement. Undisplaced fractures, or cracked ribs, are more common in athletic activity than displaced fractures, because the ribs are well stabilized by the attachment of the intercostal muscles and the fixation of each rib to its corresponding thoracic vertebra. Signs and symptoms associated with fractured ribs include localized pain which is increased with movement of the ribs, breathing deeply, coughing, and sneezing. An athlete with fractured ribs will generally refrain from breathing deeply by taking rapid shallow breaths, and may also hold the injured side in an attempt to restrict any painful movement of the chest. During gentle palpation and compression of the ribs, the athlete will indicate pain at the fracture site. If the fracture is displaced, there may also be a palpable defect in the rib and crepitation on movement or coughing. Serious complications, such as puncture of thoracic or abdominal visceral structures, can occur as a result of rib fractures.

The same mechanisms causing rib fractures may also result in **costochondral separations**. This is a separation or actual dislocation at the articulation between the rib and the cartilage connecting it to the sternum. Signs and symptoms are similar to rib fractures except the pain is localized over the costochondral junction. If the dislocation is complete, there may be a palpable defect. The athlete may also feel a click or snap as the rib dislocates and then almost immediately relocates.

Intrathoracic Injuries

Intrathoracic injuries or conditions occur very rarely during athletic activity because of the protection provided by the rib cage. However, visceral injuries can occur as the result of severe trauma to the chest or from complications accompanying a rib fracture. It is important to recognize signs and symptoms which may indicate intrathoracic involvement. Athletes who sustain an injury to the chest and exhibit any of the following should be referred to medical assistance.

1. Difficult or labored breathing
2. Shortness of breath—inability to catch breath
3. Pain increasing in chest
4. Vomiting or coughing up blood

Support of the Ribs

The main objective for support of injured ribs is to immobilize the area and protect against additional trauma. Several methods are used, such as elastic rib belts, rib jackets, elastic wraps, or tape. Figure 4-1 illustrates a method of taping injured ribs.

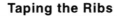

Taping the Ribs

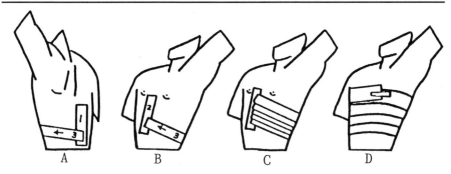

A   B   C   D

Fig. 4-1

Have the athlete stand with the arm on the affected side raised over his or her head. Place a gauze pad over the nipple if tape is to be applied over it. The athlete should be instructed to exhale before each strip of tape is applied to allow for better immobilization.

Start by applying an anchor (#1) on the uninjured rib side of the spinal column (A). An anchor (#2) in front should be applied on the uninjured rib side of the sternum (B). Strip #3 starts on the back anchor, follows the contour of the ribs (athlete exhaling) and ends on the front anchor. This strip should be applied below the injured area. Additional strips of tape overlapping one-half are applied until the injured area is covered (C). This taping procedure is locked by encircling the rib cage with elastic adhesive tape or an elastic wrap (D).

SPINE

The spine is a remarkable structure in that it can withstand tremendous stresses and forces and at the same time remain quite flexible and mobile. The spine encases and provides protection for the spinal cord. Trauma to the spine can produce devastating injuries, which can be fatal or cause irreversible damage to the spinal cord resulting in permanent paralysis.

The spine consists of 33 vertebrae, which are subdivided into seven cervical, twelve thoracic, five lumbar, five sacral (fused), and four coccygeal (fused) vertebrae (Figure 4-2). The 24 nonfused vertebrae lying superior to the sacrum increase in size from the first cervical through the fifth lumbar. Between each of these vertebrae is an intervertebral disc. Discs act as shock absorbers and allow movement between adjacent vertebrae.

Anterior View of the Spine

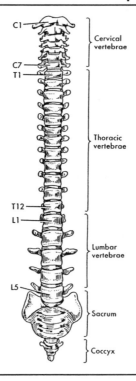

Fig. 4-2

Each intervertebral disc consists of two structures (1) the **annulus fibrosus** and (2) the **nucleus pulposus**. The annulus fibrosus is the tough outer layer that connects the bodies of adjacent vertebrae. The nucleus pulposus is the semisolid, gelatinous substance located in the center of the disc. It contains a high percentage of water (70% to 80%), which allows the disc to change shape easily during movement of the vertebral column. The intervertebral discs are subject to dehydration as a result of pressure placed on them. Minute quantities of water can be squeezed out of each disc and are absorbed into the bloodstream during a day's activity. This can result in an individual losing up to 2 cm of height during a day. During rest and sleep, when the pressure on the discs is least, water is reabsorbed from the bloodstream and original height is regained. When the nucleus pulposus herniates through the annulus fibrosus, an individual has a ruptured disc, commonly called a **slipped disc**.

As mentioned previously the spinal cord is encased within the spinal canal. This is a continuation of the motor and sensory pathways from the brain. The spinal cord is surrounded by meninges, cerebrospinal fluid, a cushion of adipose tissue, and blood vessels. The cord extends approximately 17-18 inches in the adult and is less than 1/2 inch in diameter. It is extremely sensitive to injury and damage is irreparable.

The nerves arising from the spinal cord connect the central nervous system to the rest of the body. A nerve root is that portion of the nerve that connects it to the spinal cord and is the most proximal segment of the peripheral nervous system. There are 31 pairs of spinal nerves which come off of the spinal cord. They have no special names but are merely numbered according to the level of the spinal column at which they emerge. Thus, there are eight cervical, twelve thoracic, five lumbar, five sacral, and one coccygeal pair of spinal nerves. A pair of these nerves leave the spinal column between each vertebrae and branch out to innervate the various parts of the body.

Each spinal nerve supplies sensory fibers to the areas of skin on the body surface that are arranged in a definite segmental pattern. Each strip of skin supplied by a given spinal nerve is called a **dermatome**. Although there is considerable overlap in the innervation of each dermatome, sensation in each band is associated with a particular spinal nerve; loss of sensation in a dermatome segment suggests injury to the spinal nerve supplying that segment.

Myotomes are a group of muscles innervated by a single nerve root. Because most muscles receive innervation from more than one nerve segment, only subtle motor dysfunction is usually noted with a lesion of a single nerve root. However, a lesion of a peripheral nerve may lead to complete motor dysfunction of the muscles supplied by that nerve. You should test for dermatomes and myotomes anytime nerve involvement is suspected.

INJURIES to the SPINE

Injuries involving the spine can be extremely serious including permanent paralysis or death. It is therefore imperative that you protect the athlete from further injury whenever an injury to the cervical spine is suspected. Ill-advised assessment procedures and improper handling and transporting maneuvers may cause irreparable spinal cord damage to an athlete who has suffered a spine fracture or dislocation. Therefore utmost caution must be used in evaluating, treating, and handling the athlete who has suffered an injury to the spine. This is one area of the body with which it is certainly better to be conservative and cautious rather than to risk a lifetime of paralysis, or possibly death, for the athlete.

Serious injuries of the spine, such as fractures and dislocations, are not common in athletics; however they do occur. The potential for this type of an injury is inherent in almost any sport. Football, however, provides the greatest potential for serious cervical spine injuries, as the head is often used in blocking and tackling techniques. Diving and gymnastics also provide mechanisms for devastating neck injuries. Most fatal or paralyzing injuries occur when an athlete's neck is in flexion and receiving a blow to the crown of the head, such as putting the head down and using the top of the head to make contact with an opponent. This type of mechanism can cause either a fracture or subluxations of the vertebrae, which may produce lesions to the spinal cord. The spinal cord may be completely or partially transected, contused, or concussed. A spinal cord contusion can cause edematous swelling within the cord, resulting in various degrees of temporary or permanent damage. A spinal cord concussion may cause transitory paralysis and symptoms, but complete recovery is usual. It is important to recognize signs and symptoms which may indicate severe spinal injuries and seek medical assistance immediately. Following is a list of findings which indicate an athlete has a potentially serious spinal injury and should be protected from further trauma and referred to medical assistance.

1. Paralysis—inability to move
2. Loss of normal sensations
3. Pain, tenderness, or deformity along the spinal column
4. Unremitting neck or back pain
5. Weakness noted in extremities
6. Loss of coordination of extremities
7. Unusual sensations in the extremities
8. Doubt regarding the presence of spinal cord involvement

Spine Sprains and Strains

Injuries to the spine which occur more commonly are sprains and strains, which often occur simultaneously. There are numerous ligaments and muscles attached to and acting on the spinal column. These structures are susceptible to injury due to the many types of stresses and forces subjected on the spine during athletic activity. It is often difficult to differentiate between a sprain and strain because of the complex anatomy. With either of these injuries there may be tenderness, spasm, and increased pain on active motion and stretching. Both these injuries are normally treated symptomatically. With more severe injuries there will be localized pain and muscle spasm, and the athlete may complain of an insecure feeling about the neck. Any athlete with less than a full, pain-free range of motion, persistent paresthesia (abnormal sensations), or weakness should be protected and excluded from further athletic activity. These injuries should be referred to a physician for further radiographic and neurologic evaluations.

Nerve Syndrome

Occasionally athletes will suffer a nerve syndrome, especially in the cervical area. This usually results from forced lateral flexion, causing the nerve roots to be either stretched or impinged. This is commonly known as a **pinched nerve, burner, stinger,** or **hot shot,** and is characterized by sharp, burning radiating pain. When the cervical plexus is involved, the athlete may complain of pain shooting into the posterior scalp, behind the ear, around the neck, or down the top of the shoulder. If the brachial plexus is involved, the athlete may complain of radiating pain, numbness, and loss of function of the arm and possibly the hand. Symptoms usually subside in minutes, but such injuries may leave residual soreness and burning or prickling sensations. Severe or repeated nerve syndrome episodes should be evaluated by a physician.

HEAD

Injuries involving the head and cervical spine constitute the most potentially serious of all athletic injuries. While discussed separately in this manual, head and neck injuries can occur together and result from the same mechanisms of injury. Therefore, it is important to consider both areas whenever managing an athlete with trauma to the head or neck.

Head injuries can occur in any sport and in a variety of ways. However, most head injuries are caused by the application of some type of sudden force to the head, usually a direct blow. This type of trauma may be caused by a collision or being struck. Head injuries may involve the scalp, skull, or brain.

INJURIES to the SCALP

The scalp offers considerable protection for the skull. Without this protection, the skull could be fractured or the brain injured by much less force. Injuries to the scalp may or may not involve the skull or brain. An athlete may suffer a severe brain injury without any observable trauma to the scalp; on the other hand, an athlete may have a dramatic-looking scalp injury with little or no brain damage. The true severity of head injuries may not be reflected by the appearance of scalp wounds. However, any scalp injury is indicative of forceful trauma to the head and suggests that further evaluation of the head should continue.

The most common athletic injuries to the scalp are contusions and lacerations. Because the scalp is highly vascularized and may bleed profusely if cut, scalp wounds many times appear worse than they actually are. Contusions about the scalp are marked by local tenderness and swelling. Bleeding between the skin and underlying tissue may result in a hematoma, which is commonly referred to as a "goose egg." If small blood vessels beneath the skin have been disrupted, there will be an ecchymosis in the area.

Lacerations of the scalp usually bleed quite freely and have a frightening appearance initially. The source of bleeding should be located, and the bleeding controlled by direct pressure before continuing the evaluation of the head. Remember, scalp wounds are indicative of trauma to the head and are secondary considerations to neurologic assessment of the brain and spinal cord.

INJURIES to the SKULL

The skull consists of two major divisions: the cranium, and the face. The cranium is a rigid, bony cavity encasing the brain, our master organ. Skull fractures are not common in athletics but may occur when an athlete with an unprotected head receives a severe blow. It may be very difficult to recognize a skull fracture. Bleeding or the presence of cerebrospinal fluid draining from the ear or nose may be the only indication. You must be alert to signs and symptoms which may indicate possible skull fractures. These are as follows:

1. Leakage of cerebrospinal fluid from the ears or nose
2. Discoloration over mastoid area (**Battle's sign**)
3. Discoloration under eyes (**raccoon eyes**)

INJURIES to the BRAIN

Injuries to the brain constitute the most serious threat to an athlete. These usually result from movement of the semisolid brain within the cranium. The brain, surrounded by cerebrospinal fluid, has limited freedom to move. Whenever a sudden force or impact is applied to the head, there can be an abrupt change of momentum for the brain, resulting in significant movement of the brain within the skull. This gives rise to the common mechanisms resulting in brain injury (Figure 4-3). These are (A) an agitation or shaking of the brain, (B) direct transmission of force from the skull to the underlying brain, (C) contrecoup or the brain rebounds and impacts against the side opposite the blow,

Common Mechanisms Resulting in Brain injury

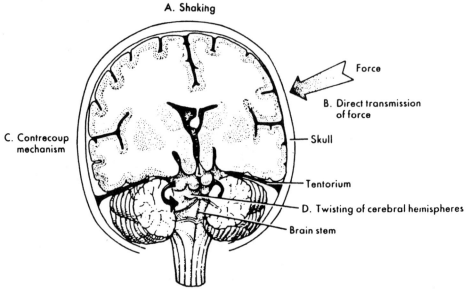

Fig. 4-3

and (D) twisting or swirling of the brain within the cranium. These mechanisms can give rise to a concussion, contusion, or additional intracranial involvement.

Concussion

The most common injury to the brain is a **concussion**. A concussion is a syndrome involving an immediate and transient impairment in the ability of the brain to function properly. Concussions are often classified into three degrees of severity according to their accompanying signs and symptoms (Table 4-1).

Mild Cerebral Concussion (first degree)— symptoms include no loss of consciousness. There may be momentary mental confusion, possible memory loss, mild ringing in the ears (tinnitus), mild dizziness and headache. There is usually no lack of coordination or unsteadiness. The athlete normally recovers quickly, with no residual symptoms. However, the athlete should be watched closely for any signs of changing orientation or additional post-concussion symptoms.

Classification of Cerebral Concussions

Signs/ Symptoms	Mild (1°)	Moderate (2°)	Severe (3°)
Consciousness	No loss, stunned, dazed	Transitory loss (up to 5 min.)	Prolonged loss (over 5 min)
Confusion	None to momentary	Slight	Severe
Memory Loss	None to slight	Mild retrograde amnesia	Prolonged retrograde amnesia
Tinnitus	Mild	Moderate	Severe
Dizziness	Mild	Moderate	Severe
Unsteadiness	Usually none	Varied	Marked

Table 4-1

Moderate Cerebral Concussion (second degree)— results in a loss of consciousness lasting less than five minutes. This is usually followed by slight mental confusion and a temporary loss of memory (amnesia). Amnesia may take the form of retrograde amnesia, in which there is a loss of memory for events that occurred before the injury, or anterograde amnesia, in which there is a loss of memory for events occurring immediately after awakening. Dizziness, ringing in the ears, unsteadiness, blurred vision, double vision, nausea, and headache are also common symptoms and may be experienced in varying combinations. The athlete usually recovers within five minutes, but may have symptoms lasting several weeks. Athletes suffering moderate concussions should be referred to medical assistance for further evaluation and follow-up care. It is important that these athletes are closely observed for 24 hours for any changes or complications.

Severe Cerebral Concussion (third degree)—prolonged loss of consciousness (over 5 minutes). This is usually followed by prolonged amnesia, mental confusion, dizziness, headache, and marked unsteadiness. The recovery rate is slow and this athlete must be referred to a physician.

Normally an athlete who has suffered a concussion will improve rapidly to an alert state of consciousness. The greatest concern for anyone who is responsible for caring for the athlete with a head injury is the possible development of intracranial involvement. The signs and symptoms of an athlete suffering from a concussion are reversible and will appear to be worse on the initial evaluation and then improve. If the signs and symptoms become progressively worse, it suggests that there is an expanding lesion within the cranium. For example, a neurologic assessment of an athlete who has a concussion should not reveal abnormalities in pupil size, movements, reflexes, sensations, strength, or respirations. Any deterioration in these neurologic signs indicate additional intracranial involvement such as hemorrhaging or swelling.

Post-Concussion Syndrome

Post-concussion syndrome consists of headache (especially with exertion), dizziness, fatigue, irritability, and impaired memory and concentration. These symptoms may persist for days or weeks and indicate altered brain functioning. These symptoms must be monitored periodically and the athlete withheld from activity as long as they persist.

Contusion

Contusions, or bruising of the brain, results when the brain impacts against the skull or is raked over bony irregularities, especially on the floor of the skull. Contusions to the hemispheres may result in a lack of nerve function of the bruised portion of the brain, but usually will not result in a loss of consciousness. Signs that suggest an athlete may have a cerebral contusion are any numbness, weakness, loss of memory, aphasia (inability to communicate), or general misbehavior when he or she is alert. An athlete with a cerebral contusion also remains stable or begins improving. Any deterioration suggests additional intracranial involvement.

Second Impact Syndrome

Second impact syndrome occurs occasionally when an athlete sustains a second head injury before symptoms associated with a previous injury have cleared. Repeated closed head injuries can predispose the brain to vascular congestion due to loss of autoregulation of the brain's blood supply. This can lead to vascular engorgement within the cranium, increased intracranial pressure, and possibly death. Second impact syndrome can occur as a result of repeated trauma that may appear to be minor compared to the original episode. Prevention is the only sure cure. Therefore, it is essential that an athlete who is symptomatic from a head injury must not be allowed to participate in contact or collision activities until all cerebral symptoms have subsided.

Intracranial Involvement

Intracranial involvement is a potentially life-threatening consequence of a head injury. This normally is the result of (1) edema (swelling) and/or (2) hemorrhaging within the cranium. Either, or a combination, of these two can lead to rapid deterioration of an athlete's condition and must be recognized if death or disability is to be averted. The same forces resulting in a concussion or contusion may also cause blood vessel damage and swelling and/or hemorrhaging. The result can cause an increased intracranial pressure, which accounts for the deteriorating signs and symptoms, such as decreasing level of consciousness, loss of movement, slowing of pupil reaction or a dilating pupil. It cannot be overemphasized how important it isto recognize an expanding intracranial lesion.

Managing Injuries to the Brain

In caring for an athlete who has had a head injury it is important to establish a neurologic baseline. This gives you and the physician a point of reference. If the athlete improves from this baseline, there is a good chance that there is no additional intracranial involvement. Remember it may take hours for these symptoms to develop. When an athlete's condition deteriorates or becomes worse than the original baseline, it suggests that intracranial involvement is developing. Information required for this neurologic baseline is as follows:

Level of Consciousness. Establishing and monitoring the level of consciousness is the most important neurologic sign to be evaluated. Question the athlete in an attempt to evaluate the level of alertness, responsiveness, awareness, and orientation. Note the initial level of consciousness and determine any subsequent changes.

In most instances, the athlete's level of consciousness will improve in a short period of time. If the athlete regains consciousness quickly, the prognosis for a rapid and uneventful recovery is good. If the athlete regains consciousness slowly, the prognosis is more guarded. The athlete who shows minimal or very slow improvement should be referred to a physician or medical facility. A decrease in the level of consciousness is the most sensitive indicator of additional intracranial involvement. Anytime the level of consciousness deteriorates, immediate medical attention is indicated.

In most instances the unconscious athlete will regain consciousness in a short period of time. However, an athlete who remains unconscious creates a difficult situation. Whenever managing an athlete who remains unconscious, there are several important points to remember.

1. Make sure they have an open airway and are breathing
2. Don't remove headgear unless absolutely necessary
3. Don't move until awake or you have medical assistance
4. Use no smelling salts or inhalants
5. Look for obvious deformities, bleeding, etc
6. Continue to monitor breathing, pulse, pupils, until the athlete regains consciousness

Headache. Headache is another frequent symptom of a head injury, and an important consideration that should be discussed while talking with an injured athlete. A headache that becomes progressively more severe is an alarming symptom that may indicate additional intracranial involvement. The persistence of a headache indicates that whatever damage occurred to the brain has not subsided, and the athlete should not return to activity. The cessation of the headache is probably the most reliable indicator that adequate recovery has occurred and the athlete can return to activity, providing also that there are no other positive neurologic signs. As you periodically check on the health status of an athlete who has suffered an injury to the head, remember to question the athlete about his or her headache.

Sensations. While questioning the athlete, inquire about any sensations they are experiencing such as pain, numbness, weakness, or tingling sensations. Does the athlete complain of ringing in the ears, dizziness, nausea, or blurred or double vision.

Pupils. It is important to check the quality and reaction of the pupils. Both pupils should be symmetric in size and react quickly and equally to light. When one pupil becomes larger and shows a decreased response to light, there is strong evidence for increased intracranial pressure. Also observe the eye movements. Normally, the eyes gaze straight ahead, unless focused on something. The movement of the eyes should be coordinated; with a head injury, the gaze may be abnormal, or the eyes may turn in different directions. Any abnormal, uncoordinated, or involuntary movement of the eyes may indicate intracranial involvement. If the athlete is conscious, instruct him or her to follow your finger with the eyes and notice whether eye movement is paralyzed or decreased in any direction.

Respirations. Observe the respiratory rate and pattern. Abnormal breathing patterns may indicate brain dysfunction and the need for medical assistance.

FACE

The face is made up of 14 bones which are largely subcutaneous and readily palpable. Facial injuries are fairly common in athletic activity. However, their frequency and severity have declined in recent years, because more sports are requiring the use of protective devices such as mouth guards, eye guards, ear guards, and face masks. Athletes in many sports, however, have no protection for the face, and a variety of facial injuries can occur. Remember, any facial injury is indicative of trauma to the head, which can also result in injuries to the brain or spinal cord. Because of the great vascularity of the face, profuse bleeding can result in dramatic-appearing injuries. Do not concentrate on facial trauma to the exclusion of possible associated injuries to the head or neck, which may be more serious.

Soft Tissue Injuries

The most common facial injuries are contusions, abrasions, and lacerations of the skin. These injuries are treated much as they would be if located anywhere else on the body; however, the need for optimal cosmetic results demands careful evaluation and care. Athletes who have isolated injuries to the skin of the face, can normally return to activity after receiving primary wound care and bleeding has been controlled. If lacerations are carefully cleaned and protected, suturing can be delayed as long as 6 hours after the primary injury. Careful inspections and palpation of the bony structures underlying lacerations, contusions, and abrasions is very important to rule out fractures of the face, nose, or skull. Any suggestion of fracture should promptly be referred to medical assistance.

Jaw Injuries

The jaw is composed of an upper jaw, or maxilla, and a lower jaw, or mandible. The mandible is the only movable bone in the skull and is the largest and strongest of the group. This bone has bony contact with the rest of the skull only at the temporomandibular (TMJ) joints and the teeth. The temporomandibular joint is the only synovial, or diarthrotic, joint of the skull and is enclosed in a thin, loose articular capsule that is weakly reinforced by support ligaments. The mandible can be elevated, depressed, protruded, retracted, and moved from side to side.

Injuries to the jaw normally occur as the result of a direct blow. Fractures to the mandible are more common than fractures to the maxilla or dislocations of the temporomandibular joint. The most common fracture of the mandible is near the angle of the lower jaw. Any contusion or suspected fracture of the mandible should be carefully palpated along the body to determine areas of point tenderness, swelling, or deformity. If there is no obvious deformity or abnormal movement observed, ask the athlete to open and close his or her mouth and appose the teeth. Does the jaw open and close normally on both sides? Do the teeth line up correctly? Palpate the temporomandibular joint as the athlete moves the jaw. If there is malocclusion of the teeth or increased pain on movement, the athlete should be referred to a physician for further assessment.

A dislocation of the temporomandibular joint does not occur very often in athletic activity. However, when it does occur, it is normally the result of a blow to the side of the jaw with the mouth open. The major signs to recognize in a temporomandibular joint dislocation are loss of jaw movement and malocclusion of the teeth. These athletes should be referred to a physician for reduction.

Nose Injuries

Nosebleeds. Hemorrhage from the nose is common in athletic facial injuries. Nosebleeds rarely become serious enough to jeopardize the life of the athlete. Because the nasal cavity is a bony space, even serious hemorrhage usually can be controlled by packing the cavity with gauze or cotton and applying pressure to the nostril of the bleeding side (Figure 4-4). Cold compresses also can be applied to the nasal area in an attempt to constrict the blood vessels.

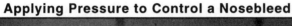

Applying Pressure to Control a Nosebleed

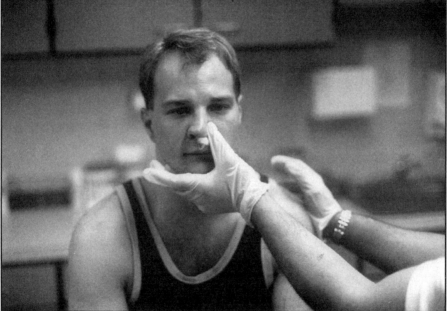

Fig. 4-4

Nasal fractures. The two nasal bones are the most frequently fractured bones in the face. These usually result from a blow to the nose and often cause bleeding which must be controlled. Nasal fractures normally exhibit tenderness at the site, deformity, swelling, and possibly crepitation. Whenever there is a question about the abnormal deviation of an injured nose, it is a good practice to allow the athlete to view his or her nose in a mirror to evaluate the normal alignment and contour. You can also look at the nasal openings from underneath to assess symmetry.

If obvious abnormal deviation is not present, the injured area should be gently palpated. Carefully feel the two nasal bones between your thumb and forefingers to locate the areas of pain and tenderness. Palpation may also reveal deformity, increased mobility, or crepitation. All obvious and suspected nasal fractures should be promptly referred to a physician for further evaluation and reduction of the fracture.

Ear Injuries

Eardrum perforations. Traumatic rupture of the eardrum can be caused by the penetration of a sharp object or sudden blow across the ear. Such injuries may be characterized by sharp pain, slight hearing impairment, and ringing in the ear. Ruptured eardrums normally heal spontaneously but should be under a physician's care.

Cauliflower ear. Repeated contusions and friction-type stresses to the external ear may result in a hematoma formation between the skin and underlying cartilage. If this hematoma remains untreated, it turns to scar tissue and can only be removed surgically. This can be avoided by timely aspiration of the hematoma and initiation of compression. Cauliflower ears can usually be prevented if athletes in sports such as wrestling will use their headgear.

Swimmer's ear. Swimmer's ear is a common infection of the external ear in athletes. It can be either bacterial or fungal in origin and is usually associated with prolonged exposure to water or excessive moisture. This condition is particularly prevalent in hot, humid climates, and during the summer. The S-shaped auditory canal is designed to protect the ear against invasion by foreign objects but also prevents water from escaping. This retained moisture is the main predisposing factor in most cases of swimmer's ear. The infection generally involves the auditory canal and perhaps the auricle. Ear pain is the most common symptom of swimmer's ear. In early stages the pain is usually mild and may be accompanied by itching. In later stages, pain can be severe and there may be a discharge from the ear. The ear as a whole is tender, and pressure may cause pain. The canal is red and swollen. The athlete may report a feeling of "fullness" in the ear. Swimmer's ear generally responds quickly to treatment. Early referral to a physician is recommended. Any treatment routine should include prevention techniques so that athletes, who spend long hours in the water, learn to care for their ears to avoid recurring infections.

Teeth Injuries

Athletic related dental injuries have decreased over the years as a result of the use of mouth guards and face masks. However, dental injuries still occur, particularly in those sports that do not require mouth protection. It is important for you to know the proper techniques of caring for dental injuries to prevent the loss of permanent teeth or later complications. This is especially true when teeth are displaced from their normal position or knocked out of the mouth. The extent of trauma involved in dental injuries can be difficult to assess because the injury may not be readily visible.

The first step in evaluating a dental injury is to locate the source of bleeding. Use a gauze pad to wipe away most of the blood around the teeth, gums, and lips. If there is little or no bleeding from the soft tissues and the seepage of blood seems to be coming from around the tooth, the tooth may be injured. Test the tooth by applying mild finger pressure inward and outward (Figure 4-5). If the movement of the tooth is similar to surrounding teeth and the tooth is not painful, numb, or fractured, the bleeding probably involves only the gum tissues sur-

Applying Mild Finger Pressure to an Injured Tooth

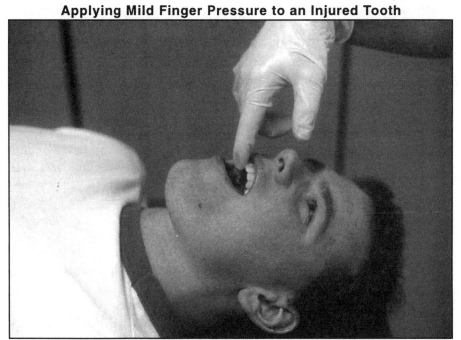

Fig. 4-5

rounding the tooth. If the tooth is painful, numb, or seems depressed, the athlete should be referred to a dentist. If these symptoms are not expressed by the athlete, he or she can resume activity provided no further care is required for any soft tissue injuries.

If a tooth is loosened and shifted in the bone, the blood supply may be compromised. Within months this tooth may turn grey and require a root canal. Teeth that have shifted should be quickly repositioned by firm finger pressure and referred to a dentist. If dental referral and proper treatment is delayed longer than 24 hours, the tooth may eventually turn grey.

If there is a small corner fracture or chip off a tooth that is not sensitive to air when the athlete inhales vigorously, athletic activity can continue. However, if the fracture is sufficient enough to expose the dentin, it is usually sensitive to air, unless numbed by the trauma. Inspect the broken tooth carefully to see if the fracture cuts across the tip of the pulp or if the pink pulp is visible. If the pulp is exposed, the athlete should receive immediate dental treatment. If the pulp is not exposed but the tooth is sensitive to air, the athlete may be permitted to continue activity as he or she desires. Tooth injuries that are sensitive to air should be referred to dental treatment within 2 to 3 hours after the trauma. An athlete who exhibits a severe fracture of a tooth should be referred to dental treatment immediately.

Any tooth that is knocked out intact (avulsed) should be saved, cleaned, and either put back into the socket or transported with the athlete to a dentist as soon as possible. Dental research has shown that almost any avulsed tooth can be replanted and retained if the ligamentous components of the tooth are kept viable. When a tooth is avulsed, half of the periodontal ligament remains in the socket and half remains attached to the tooth. The portion that remains in the socket continues to be viable because it is bathed in a pool of blood that fills the socket. The problem area is the portion of the ligament which remains on the tooth root. If this portion remains viable, it will reattach to the periodontal ligament fibers remaining in the socket when replanted. Treatment must therefore center on maintaining the viability of the periodontal ligament still attached to the tooth. The best possible method of creating this environment is by placing the tooth back in the socket immediately. If replanted within 15-30 minutes, there is a 90% chance of saving the tooth. After this time, the periodontal ligament cells may have dried out and successful reattachment diminishes rapidly. If the tooth is not replanted at the scene, the success rate of saving the tooth is almost totally dependent upon how the tooth is stored, preserved, and handled.

Do not touch the tooth on the root portion as the cells can be crushed and destroyed. The avulsed tooth must not be allowed to dry out and should be kept in a medium compatible with the ligament cells. There are Emergency Tooth Preserving Systems on the market and should be required in every training room. These kits contain a solution to store the avulsed tooth which can keep the cells viable for 4-12 hours. These solutions do not require refrigeration and can be kept on the shelf for long periods of time. Saliva can be used as a storage medium for short periods of time (less than one hour). Milk is an acceptable storage medium for short periods of time, providing it is available, cold and whole. Powdered, skim, or sour milk are damaging to the periodontal ligament. Sterile saline is also damaging to the tooth cells if the avulsed tooth is allowed to soak in it for more than 1 hour. Avoid allowing the tooth to dry out or soak in tap water. The athlete should be referred to a dentist as soon as possible. X-rays should be taken within 24 to 48 hours to rule out a fracture and follow-up films should be taken within one to three months.

Eye Injuries

Significant numbers of sports-related eye injuries occur as a result of head or facial trauma. Increased popularity and participation in tennis and racquetball, for example, have resulted in a dramatic increase in the number of eye contusion injuries. Most of these injuries could be prevented by wearing protective eye wear and following a few safety rules. The use of eye protection should be encouraged whenever possible. When an eye injury does occur, a basic knowledge of ocular assessment techniques permits rapid screening of eye injuries or related complaints and will facilitate referral of the athlete to medical assistance when required.

Foreign bodies and abrasions. Among the more common conditions of the eye to be managed during athletic activity are foreign bodies and abrasions. Athletes often express the feeling of having something in the eye. It is important to know that foreign bodies in the eye and abrasion injuries of the conjunctiva and cornea produce almost identical symptoms, that is, pain, increased tearing, and the sensation of something in the eye. Superficial foreign bodies can be removed with a moistened cotton-tipped applicator or irrigating solution. If no foreign body can be located, the presence of an abrasion should be suspected and, if symptoms continue, the athlete should be referred to a physician. Athletes who have suffered a corneal abrasion will continue to insist that something is in the eye.

Lacerations. Minor lacerations to the skin of the eyelid that do not involve the lid margin are generally not serious. If the margin of the eyelid is cut, the injury is much more serious. All lacerations that involve either the upper or lower lid margin should be referred to an ophthalmologist. Such lacerations may cut through the tarsal plate and lead to a "notched" lid, which can be disfiguring. In addition, persistent and troublesome tearing can also result from lacerations that cut the lid margin.

Any laceration of the eyeball itself is a serious injury with potentially grave consequences. The athlete will usually complain of pain in the eye and decreased vision. In looking at the eye, you may see the corneal laceration, or the pupil may appear tear-shaped. If a laceration of the eyeball is noted, further examination in this area should stop. Reassure the athlete and refer him or her immediately to an ophthalmologist after placing a protective pad or shield over the eye. Often it is helpful to cover both eyes at the same time to reduce eyemovement and lower the likelihood of further irritation. Do not exert any pressure on the eye.

Conjunctivitis. Conjunctivitis is an inflammation or infection of the conjunctiva, the membrane covering the anterior eyeball and inner surface of the eyelids. There can be a number of causes including bacteria, viruses, chemicals, and allergies. Symptoms include redness of the eye, a foreign body sensation, and fullness of the eyelids. There may be some itching and the eyelids may be stuck together on awakening. Physical examination signs include redness of the eye, tearing, some discharge, and swelling of the eyelids.

Blunt-blow injuries. Contusion types of injuries can occur to the eye, especially in sports such as racquetball and handball. This trauma frequently results in a black eye (**periorbital contusion**) or red eye (**subconjunctival hemorrhage**, which is blood in the white of the eyeball). Hemorrhage into the anterior chamber of the eye following a blunt blow is called **hyphema**. Assessment of this condition is usually no problem because the blood can be seen through the cornea as it collects in a pool in the lower portion of the anterior chamber of the eye. The athlete may also complain of pain in the eye and fuzzy vision. Although this condition clears spontaneously in almost all cases, referral to a physician is required because of the possibility of secondary hemorrhage.

A serious injury that can result from blunt-blow trauma to the eye is called an **orbital blow-out fracture**. If the eye has been subjected to a severe blunt blow (such as a baseball or hockey puck injury), the possibility of a fractured orbit should always be considered. In blow-out fractures, the floor of the orbit is pushed into the maxillary sinus. As a result of the fracture, the mobility of the affected eye is restricted. This occurs because the ocular muscles are often trapped or pinched at the fracture site. If there is restriction of eye movement (especially an inability to look upward), or if the athlete complains of double vision following a severe blunt-blow injury to the eye or face, an orbital fracture should be considered. In most cases of orbital fracture, multiple and potentially serious eye injuries occur. Referral to an ophthalmologist is essential.

Displaced contact lenses. The use of contact lenses by athletes has greatly increased and presents some problems for the coach. Hard contact lenses are more likely than the newer soft lenses to cause eye abrasions, slip around, pop out, and become lost. The coach may be involved with locating and recentering displaced contact lenses. To care for an athlete wearing contact lenses, wetting solution, lens cases, and a mirror should be available.

INJURIES TO THE UPPER EXTREMITIES

This unit will be concerned with the more common athletic injuries or conditions involving the upper extremities. Upper extremity injuries occur less frequently than injuries to the lower extremities. However, the upper extremities play a vital role in most types of athletic activity and the proper management of injuries to this area of the body is very important.

SHOULDER

The shoulder is more than simply the articulation of the arm with the torso. It encompasses all of the intricate anatomical and functional relationships between the thorax, clavicle, scapula, and humerus. This area is usually referred to as the shoulder girdle or complex. Each portion plays an important role in the coordinated movements of the arm. An athletic injury to any one area of the shoulder may impair function of the whole unit.

The anatomical structures of the shoulder girdle are illustrated in Figure 5-1. There are three joints or articulations which make up this area of the body, the sternoclavicular, acromioclavicular, and glenohumeral joints.

Right Shoulder - anterior view

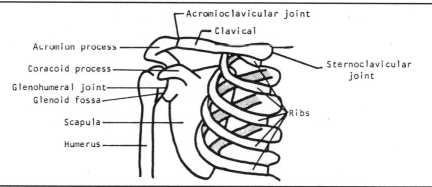

Fig. 5-1

STERNOCLAVICULAR JOINT

The sternoclavicular joint is the only bony attachment between the upper limb and the axial skeleton. The articulation between the clavicle and sternum is actually the pivot point about which movements of the shoulder occur. Athletic injuries involving this joint occur infrequently.

Sternoclavicular Sprains

The most common injuries to the sternoclavicular joint are sprains. These result when force is directed along the long axis of the clavicle. When supporting ligaments are stretched significantly or torn, the sternal end of the clavicle may dislocate. This dislocation is almost always anteriorly. The injury commonly results in tenderness, swelling, and a visible prominence at the sternoclavicular joint. Athletes suffering a complete dislocation of the sternoclavicular joint are frequently placed in a brace or taped to immobilize the area for three to five weeks.

Clavicular Injuries

Injuries involving the clavicle are fairly common in athletics. Because the bone is subcutaneous, it is subjected to contusions caused by any type of direct trauma to the area. Contusions will cause tenderness and swelling at the site of injury but normally little increase in pain with shoulder motion.

The clavicle is also frequently fractured during athletic activity. This is especially true of preadolescent and adolescent athletes. In older athletes, ligament injuries to the sternoclavicular or acromioclavicular joint are more likely to occur than fractures. Most fractured clavicles in young athletes are of the **greenstick** type, which can be difficult to recognize because there is no displacement evident. Suspect a greenstick fracture whenever there is tenderness over the shaft of the clavicle in a young athlete who has suffered trauma to the area. In older athletes the fracture is usually complete and the medial fragment is more prominent.

ACROMIOCLAVICULAR JOINT

The acromioclavicular joint is the articulation between the lateral end of the clavicle and the acromion process of the scapula. This small synovial joint permits numerous gliding movements. The ligaments supporting this joint are richly supplied with sensory nerves, so an injury to this area is usually quite painful.

Acromioclavicular Sprains

Injuries to the acromioclavicular joint are common in athletics. They generally result from a blow to the tip of the shoulder which drives the acromion downward, or falling on an outstretched arm, which can drive the acromion backward and away from the clavicle. Either of these mechanisms can cause a sprain of the supporting ligaments, an injury commonly called a **shoulder separation**. An athlete suffering an acromioclavicular sprain will generally exhibit varying degrees of tenderness, swelling, instability and an increase in pain with any effort to stress the joint. A third-degree sprain will usually show an upward riding clavicle in relation to the acromion. A chronic separated shoulder has traditionally been called a **knocked-down shoulder**.

Shoulder separations are generally treated like any other sprain type of injuries. Most second degree separations require immobilization for a period of weeks for fibrous healing to take place. Third degree separations often result in corrective surgery. When returning to activity the area needs to be supported and protected. This can be accomplished with a protective pad and a combination of wrapping or taping. Wrapping using the shoulder spica was discussed previously. A method of stabilizing the acromioclavicular joint with tape is illustrated later in Figure 5-2.

SHOULDER JOINT

The shoulder joint is a ball-and-socket type formed by the **glenoid fossa** of the scapula and the head of the humerus; thus called the glenohumeral joint. The large rounded head of the humerus fits into the much smaller and shallow glenoid cavity, which explains why this joint has a great range of motion, but is inherently unstable. In fact, the shoulder is considered our most mobile joint. The stability of the shoulder joint is provided mainly by the surrounding muscles. A group of muscles which are very important to the strength of the shoulder, are called the **rotator cuff muscles**, which are the (1) supraspinatus, (2) infraspinatus, (3) teres minor, and (4) subscapularis. These four muscles, also called the SITS muscles, blend with and strengthen the articular capsule, and provide significant stability to the shoulder. A detailed explanation of the complex array of movements and muscles about the shoulder girdle is beyond the scope of this manual.

INJURIES TO THE SHOULDER COMPLEX

Because of the extensive motion available and the inherent instability of the shoulder, this area of the body is very vulnerable to acute athletic injuries as well as chronic overuse conditions. The mechanisms causing most injuries are (1) direct trauma, (2) throwing movements, and (3) indirect trauma transmitted to the shoulder, such as falling on an outstretched arm.

Contusions

The most common contusion about the shoulder is to the tip of the shoulder or acromion process. This is commonly called a **shoulder pointer**. With this injury you must be concerned with a more serious injury to the acromioclavicular joint.

The deltoid muscle is also susceptible to direct blows, which can result in a contusion to the area. A possible complication of repeated contusions to this area, is the development of a bony spur sometimes referred to as a **blocker's spur** since it is seen more often in football. Like other areas of the body, contusions require protective padding when the athlete returns to activity.

Strains

A common injury about the shoulder joint is some type of muscular or musculotendinous strain. The glenohumeral joint relies on the surrounding musculature for most of its stability as well as its motion and power. Therefore the muscles and musculotendinous structures are involved in many types of athletic injuries. Various mechanisms can produce injuries to the musculotendinous units, including over-stretching, violent contractions, and repetitive use.

Strains about the shoulder are especially common in athletic activities that require the arm to propel an object, such as pitching, or to overcome a resistance, such as in swimming. During racquet sports the shoulder serves as the fulcrum for the arm, and major stresses are placed on the elbow and forearm. However, significant and often injurious forces are also placed on the shoulder joint. Each sport presents its own problems or situations for the shoulder, and the responses to stress vary in intensity and location. The nature of shoulder strains is influenced by many things, such as the age and maturity of the athlete; the type and weight of the object being propelled; the type of delivery; the presence of weakness, fatigue, or incoordination; fibrous scarring or degenerative changes from previous injuries; and microtrauma from repetitive activity. All of these factors must be considered during the assessment of shoulder injuries.

Rotator cuff strains. Injuries involving the rotator cuff muscles may be difficult to detect and isolate because these muscles lie deep in the shoulder. Any of the mechanisms previously discussed can cause an injury to these muscles; however, when they occur in young athletes the problem is normally the result of direct trauma. As an athlete becomes older, he or she is more susceptible to rotator cuff injuries resulting from repeated stress. Repetitive use of the shoulder can result in microscopic damage to the rotator cuff muscles. A great deal of difficulty may be encountered in assessing these soft tissue lesions. Bursitis, tendinitis, partial rotator cuff tears, loose pieces of fibrocartilage, and calcific deposits are all capable of producing similar signs and symptoms.

Biceps strain. Another relatively common strain in the shoulder occurs to the long head of the biceps tendon. This is especially true in athletes who are skiing, throwing overhand, or playing tennis. The long head of the biceps tendon lies in a tubular sheath as it passes through the bicipital groove. Repetitive motion of the shoulder causes this tendon to slide up and down through the tunnel. The irritation of constant motion can cause an inflammatory reaction to develop. This bicipital tenosynovitis, sometimes called a "glass arm," will cause tenderness along the bicipital groove and pain on active and resistive contraction or passive stretching of the biceps.

Impingement syndrome. A common injury involving the soft tissues of the shoulder comprise the subacromial space and are normally referred to as an impingement syndrome. Often it begins as a tendinitis especially involving the supraspinatus or biceps tendons. As time progresses, the subdeltoid bursa becomes involved (subdeltoid bursitis). Secondary changes such as scarring, thickening of the involved tendon, chronic inflammation, and irritation of the overlying bursa frequently develop. These factors decrease the distance between the supraspinatus tendon and the acromion process, which can cause pain and crepitus as the involved tissues are squeezed or impinged between the humerus and the acromion.

Activities involving repetitive use of the arm above the horizontal level, such as throwing, tennis, or swimming (**swimmer's shoulder**), may produce this overuse syndrome. The most significant symptom of impingement is pain about the acromion, often described as "deep" within the shoulder. Initially the pain may be a dull ache about the shoulder after strenuous activity and often at night. This pain may progress to discomfort during activity and eventually affects performance. Athletes may restrict movements and refrain from particular maneuvers that cause the impingement. Physical findings include palpable tenderness over the greater tuberosity at the supraspinatus insertion, palpable tenderness along the anterior edge of the acromion, a painful arc of abduction between 60° to 120°, and pain during passive stress tests involving forced flexion and/or internal rotation of the proximal humerus.

Dislocations

Because of its inherent instability, the shoulder joint has the highest incidence of dislocations of any major joint in the body. Shoulder dislocations are classified depending on the location of the head of the humerus. The anterior, or subcoracoid dislocation is by far the most common. The mechanism of injury is forced abduction and external rotation. The athlete generally has the shoulder in an abducted, externally rotated position and receives a blow somewhere along the extremity. If the force is insufficient to cause complete dislocation, the humeral head may sublux and then relocate, causing a sprain to the anterior capsule and supporting ligaments. The athlete will often relate that the arm was forced into external rotation and abduction and he or she felt the humerus "slip out of place." This will be accompanied by pain in the anterior aspect of the joint, which is increased by any attempt to abduct and externally rotate the arm.

Dislocations of the shoulder have a high incidence of recurrence without a period of immobilization and a vigorous rehabilitation program. When a shoulder is not rehabilitated sufficiently following a dislocation, this joint is very susceptible to repeated episodes. Each successive dislocation requires less force to drive the humeral head out of the glenoid and also causes it to reduce more easily. Recurrent episodes can develop into a condition in which the shoulder will dislocate during abduction and external rotation without much additional trauma. This demonstrates the importance of early recognition and proper rehabilitation of all shoulder dislocations.

Other Conditions of the Shoulder

Adhesive capsulitis. Adhesive capsulitis, often referred to as a "frozen shoulder," is an inflammation about the rotator cuff and capsular area that can result in dense adhesions and capsular contracture causing restriction of motion and pain. The exact cause remains unknown. The onset of symptoms are often insidious with gradual increase in pain and decrease in motion. It can develop because an athlete protects a painful shoulder by limiting movement. In some cases it may develop if the joint is immobilized after a serious injury. The main feature of adhesive capsulitis is lack of passive ROM, especially rotation and abduction.

Brachial plexus injuries. Injuries to the brachial plexus normally involve the cervical spine, but the symptoms are exhibited in the shoulder and upper extremity. When an athlete's neck is violently forced into rotation or lateral flexion, especially while the opposite shoulder is depressed, considerable tension can be placed on the nerve branches of the brachial plexus. Occasionally part of the brachial plexus is compressed between the clavicle and first rib. Both of these mechanisms can result in transitory paralysis of the arm, with numbness or a burning sensation radiating down the arm and sometimes into the hand. This normally disappears in a matter of seconds to a few minutes. Occasionally recovery may take days. An injury to the brachial plexus is frequently called a "pinched nerve," "burner," "hot shot," or "stinger." Occasionally a persistent disability may result from this type of injury.

Athletes experiencing repeated episodes of brachial plexus injuries or who complain of weakness or numbness in the arm that persists for an hour or more after the injury should be carefully evaluated and referred to a physician for a neurologic examination.

Shoulder Support

Returning to activity following some type of shoulder injury, the athlete will often require some form of shoulder protection and support. Protection is often provided by a protective pad held in place with an elastic wrap such as the shoulder spica. Support is often provided by the use of an elastic wrap or taping procedure designed to limit painful motion. In addition, various types of shoulder harnesses or braces can be used to restrict painful motion. Remember, because the shoulder relies on the muscular system for much of its strength and stability, it is important that a good rehabilitation program designed at strengthening these muscles be initiated and continued.

Shoulder Taping

Figure 5-2 illustrates a common method of taping for support of the shoulder designed to restrict painful movement of the arm. Two disadvantages of using tape are irritation to the skin and difficulty in locking or holding the tape in position.

The athlete stands with the hand of the injured side resting on his or her hip. Start the taping procedure by applying two anchor strips, one around the upper arm (#1) and the second over the shoulder near the neck (#2). The anchor around the upper arm should not be overlapped as it may become constrictive. Strip #3 starts on the front of the arm anchor, is firmly pulled up over the shoulder, and ends on the top anchor (A). Strip #4 starts on the back of the arm anchor, is firmly pulled up over the shoulder, and ends on the top anchor. The two strips should form an "X" over the point of the shoulder.

Basketweave strips should be applied until the shoulder is covered, as shown in (B). The number of basketweave strips applied depends upon the amount of motion you wish to limit. For example, the more strips of tape applied down the front of the shoulder, the less backward arm motion the athlete will have.

Taping for Support of the Shoulder

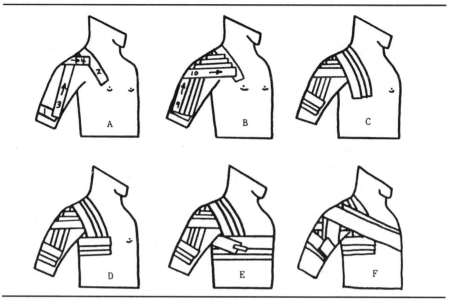

Fig. 5-2

As previously mentioned, one of the problems with taping the shoulder is locking the support strips in place. In fact, it may take more tape to lock down than it does to provide support. Figure 5-2 (C), illustrates applying lock strips over the shoulder and around the arm. If tape is applied over the nipple, it should be covered with a gauze pad. There are several techniques which will further help to lock down a basic shoulder taping. You can apply strips of tape partially around the chest (D), or elastic tape or wrap completely around the chest (E). It is also helpful to apply a shoulder spica over the tape procedure to help lock it in position (F).

ELBOW AND FOREARM

The elbow and forearm are important functional links between the shoulder and the intricate mechanisms of the hand. The elbow joint allows the arm to flex and extend, whereas the articulations between the radius and ulna permit the forearm to rotate, that is, pronate and supinate. In addition, all the extrinsic muscles of the hand originate about the elbow or forearm. Therefore, the ability to perform athletic skills involving the upper extremities is dependent on the integrity of the bones, ligaments, and muscles of the elbow and forearm.

There are really three joints about the elbow: (1) between the humerus and ulna, (2) between the humerus and radius, and (3) between the radius and ulna. Identify these joints on Figure 5-3. The elbow joint proper (humeroulnar) is a hinge joint allowing only flexion and extension. The bony projections on the distal end of the humerus, are called the medial and lateral epicondyles. The medial epicondyle is the point of attachment for the **common flexor tendon**, which is the shared tendon for the wrist flexor muscles. The lateral epicondyle is the point of attachment for the **common extensor tendon**, which is the shared tendon for the wrist extensors. These are frequent sites of athletic related trauma discussed under strains. The large bony projection on the proximal ulna, the **olecranon**, or tip of the elbow, is the point of attachment for the triceps muscle.

Right Elbow and Forearm (posterior view)

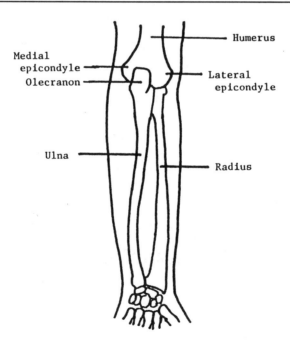

Fig. 5-3

The bones of the forearm are the ulna located on the medial (little finger) side and the radius on the lateral (thumb) side. These two bones articulate (pivot) at the proximal and distal ends allowing the movements of pronation and supination. This rotating motion occurs as the radius crosses over the stationary ulna.

INJURIES TO THE ELBOW AND FOREARM

Injuries involving the elbow and forearm are common in athletic activity. Many different types of force and stress are applied about the elbow during the various activities involved in different sports. A variety of athletic injuries can result from direct trauma to the area, indirect trauma such as falling on an outstretched hand, or acute and chronic stresses associated with throwing and swinging activities. As a group, athletic injuries to the elbow are potentially serious because inappropriate treatment may lead to functional impairment or permanent disability. Of all the large joints in the body, the elbow is the most susceptible to loss of motion after injury.

Contusions

Contusions are common injuries to this area of the body and may involve the muscles of the forearm or the subcutaneous bony prominences of the elbow. An athlete's forearms absorb the brunt of many impacts during athletic activity, especially during contact sports. Direct blows to these muscular areas can result in bruising and subsequent bleeding, producing stiffness during function and active range of motion.

Olecranon bursitis. A common injury resulting from a blow to the tip of the elbow is olecranon bursitis. Acute bursitis occurs when a blow to the tip of the elbow results in hemorrhaging into the olecranon bursa. This can cause immediate dramatic swelling, pain, and restriction of motion. Often an acute olecranon bursitis will spontaneously subside. Chronic trauma or repeated bruising to the tip of the elbow can result in the formation of excess bursal fluid with tenderness and varying amounts of swelling over the olecranon. Occasionally there will be a small palpable mass in this area. This is normally fibrous tissue but may be mistaken for a chip of bone.

Ulnar nerve contusion. An injury that almost everyone has suffered is a contusion to the ulnar nerve. As this nerve passes behind the medial epicondyle, it lies subcutaneously. A direct blow to this area may cause pain and burning sensations shooting down the ulnar side of the forearm to the ring and little finger. This is commonly referred to as "hitting the crazy bone." The pain and burning sensations are normally transient and disappear in a few minutes.

Strains

Strains to the muscular and musculotendinous structures about the elbow are common athletic injuries. These normally occur as a result of tremendous stresses being placed on the elbow joint, especially in those sports requiring throwing or swinging motions. Strains are divided into acute and chronic types. Acute strains occur when a sudden overload is applied to the contractile units of the elbow joint. Chronic strains commonly occur about the elbow as the result of continued overuse of a musculotendinous unit, with ultimate failure or impairment of function. Overuse, especially in sports requiring throwing or swinging, may cause irritation of the muscle fibers, resulting in microscopic tears of the contractile unit. Continued trauma to this area can develop into overuse syndromes and chronic degenerative processes. Chronic strains commonly occur in the region of the medial and lateral epicondyles of the humerus, depending on the muscle groups irritated. For example, overuse of the wrist flexor-pronator muscles may cause symptoms over the medial epicondyle, whereas chronic irritation of the wrist extensor-supinator muscles may result in symptoms over the lateral epicondyle. Names are frequently given to these overuse conditions depending on the athletic activity involved in at the time of their development, for example, "tennis elbow," "pitcher's elbow," or "golfer's elbow."

Little league elbow is a term used to describe elbow lesions that result from the repetitive act of throwing in immature athletes. The most common problem of the little leaguer is an injury to the epiphysis of the medial epicondyle of the humerus. This epiphysis is normally the last epiphyseal center to close around the elbow and one of the weakest. The symptoms may be of acute or gradual onset. When the onset is sudden, the injury is more likely to involve an avulsion of the epicondyle. Acute pain and tenderness over the epicondyle indicates that an immature athlete should be referred to a physician for further assessment. More commonly, little league elbow is a chronic condition, and the symptoms are usually those of persistent discomfort and stiffness about the elbow and are aggravated by use of the arm.

Sprains

Sprains of the elbow joint are moderately common in athletic activity. Because of the configuration of the ulna in the trochlear notch, this is a relatively stable joint. Injuries involving the ligamentous system of the elbow most commonly result from partial dislocations or subluxations. The mechanism of injury is frequently forced hyperextension or lateral motion. Athletes with this type of history will often describe a "click" or "pop" along with sharp pain at the time of injury. In addition to tenderness at the site of injury, there is normally localized swelling and pain on any attempt to reproduce the mechanism of injury. Pain is usually relieved by bending the elbow, and athletes will normally hold their injured extremity in some degree of flexion.

Dislocations

Dislocations involving the elbow joint are not common but can be a serious injury. The most common type of dislocation is the posterior displacement of the ulna and radius in relationship to the humerus. This normally occurs because of a fall on an outstretched hand with the elbow in extension. As the elbow is forced into hyperextension, the olecranon process is levered against the humerus, which can force the ulna backward. Elbow dislocations that remain displaced appear deformed, with the olecranon process abnormally prominent and the athlete expressing considerable pain. All elbow dislocations should be properly immobilized and referred to a physician immediately.

Fractures

Fractures about the elbow and forearm can result from any of the injury-producing mechanisms described in this unit. Normally fractures occur as the result of either direct trauma to the forearm or elbow or indirect stresses transmitted through the upper extremity as the result of falling on an outstretched arm. In addition, excessive forces associated with throwing and swinging activities may cause an interruption in bony continuity. Fractures about the elbow are among the most frequent involving children and skeletally immature athletes. Many of these involve the epiphysis because the ligamentous structures in young athletes are much stronger than the bony and cartilaginous components of the growth plate. Therefore you should maintain a high level of suspicion concerning fractures whenever evaluating an acute elbow injury in a young athlete. Fortunately, fractures of the elbow are not common in skeletally mature athletes. All epiphyses at the elbow are fused by 18 years of age.

Fractures of the forearm are common in young athletes. They are usually caused by a direct blow or falling on an outstretched hand. The signs and symptoms of forearm fractures may include point tenderness, swelling, angulation of the bone, pain on motion, disability, and crepitation. Whenever a fracture is suspected, the athlete should be referred to a physician.

Elbow Support

Frequently an injured elbow needs protection or support when the athlete returns to activity. Protection is usually offered in the form of a protective pad or elbow pad. Support is often provided by the use of adhesive tape. Most often the support is to restrict hyperextension, preventing the elbow from overextending since this is the range of motion most painful. Figure 5-4 illustrates a common method of taping to restrict hyperextension.

Taping the Elbow

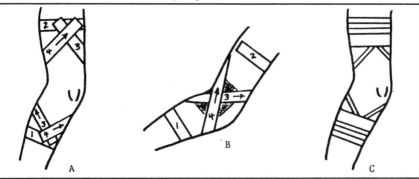

Fig. 5-4

With the elbow in a flexed position, place a gauze pad in front of the joint to prevent irritation from the tape. Anchor strips of tape (#1 and #2) ar e applied above and below the elbow joint. The anchor around the upper arm should not completely encircle the arm, as it may become constricting during activity. Strips #3 and #4 start below and behind the elbow, continue diagonally across the front of the joint, and finish above and behind the elbow (A & B).

Additional diagonal strips are applied directly over strips #3 and #4, the number of strips depending upon the severity of the injury and the athletes preference. Circular strips of tape should be applied above and below the elbow joint to lock this taping procedure (C). Again do not overlap these strips as the tape may become too constrictive. An elastic wrap or elastic tape may be applied over the tape to further secure the procedure.

WRIST AND HAND

The wrist is that area of articulation between the forearm and hand. The hand, which includes the fingers and thumb, is a functionally intricate and complex anatomical structure located at the end of our upper extremity. Precise functioning of the hand and wrist is essential to almost every type of athletic activity. Together they permit an incredible array of intricate movements and also serve to absorb or transmit forces caused by falls or traumatic contact. Because the hand and wrist normally do not bear our weight and because injuries to this area are not usually totally disabling, there is a tendency by some athletes to underestimate the severity and importance of these injuries. If neglected or unrecognized, injuries to the hand and wrist can develop into long term impairment and possibly permanent disability or disfigurement.

The wrist contains the carpal bones, the distal ends of the radius and ulna, and the proximal ends of the metacarpal bones (Figure 5-5). The bony anatomy of the hand consists of five metacarpals and 14 phalanges. There are many joints and muscles or muscle insertions within the hand which make it possible to perform a great variety of complicated movements.

Right Hand (posterior view)

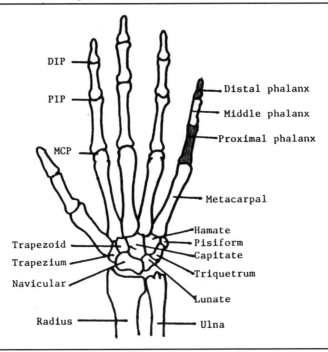

DIP

PIP

MCP

Distal phalanx

Middle phalanx

Proximal phalanx

Metacarpal

Hamate

Trapezoid — Pisiform

Trapezium — Capitate

Navicular — Triquetrum

Lunate

Radius — Ulna

Fig. 5-5

INJURIES TO THE WRIST

The wrist is a frequently injured area of the body. Athletic injuries often result from a direct blow to the wrist or stresses that force the wrist beyond its normal range of motion. The wide range of mobility available at the wrist contributes a great deal to overall hand function. The wide use of the hands in athletics, such as breaking a fall, warding off another player, grasping, catching, throwing, or hitting, frequently force the wrist beyond its normal range of motion.

Strains

Each of the many tendons that cross the wrist may be strained. This is especially true of the wrist flexors and extensors. Strains can result from a violent muscular contraction against resistance, an over-stretching such as that associated with hyperflexion or hyperextension, or chronic overuse. These injuries can also be confused with a wrist sprain or carpal fracture. Strains, however, will cause increased pain on active and resistive contraction of the muscles involved.

Wrist ganglion. Another condition that can involve the tendinous sheath or synovial joint capsule is a synovial hernia or knot-like mass called a wrist ganglion, which occurs most often on the back of the wrist. It is believed that a ganglion of this type results from a defect in the fibrous sheath of a tendon or joint, which permits a portion of the underlying synovium to herniate through it. This herniated sac forms a cystic enlargement that gradually fills with fluid and may become quite large. In athletics, this condition usually follows a strain or sprain of the wrist but can occur without any trauma. A ganglion generally appears as a small nodule over the dorsum of the wrist, but can also occur on the palmar aspect. Its cystic-like mass may vary in consistency from very soft to firm and is generally not painful. A ganglion that is painful or limits motion should be examined by a physician.

Sprains

Many athletic injuries to the wrist are sprains. They are normally caused by hyperextension or hyperflexion which stress the supporting ligaments. Always evaluate wrist sprains for a possible wrist fracture, since the symptoms will be very similar. Tenderness over the carpals or styloid processes of the radius or ulna should be referred to a physician for x-ray. If initial radiographs are negative, the athlete should be treated as if there is a sprain. In the presence of persistent pain and swelling lasting for two to three weeks a second x-ray should be requested.

Fractures

Fractures about the wrist most commonly result from forced hyperextension such as falling on an outstretched hand. This mechanism transmits the force of the fall through the capitate and navicular (scaphoid) bones, to the radius. The navicular is the most commonly fractured of all carpals because of its size and location. This bone is an oval, elongated bone with a narrowed central portion. It is this area that is most vulnerable to fracture. A fractured navicular will cause pain just distal to the radius, and point tenderness in the **anatomical** snuffbox. The anatomical snuffbox is formed by tendons of the thumb and becomes prominent when the thumb is extended. The navicular lies just below this indentation and can be felt upon palpation. All wrist injuries exhibiting tenderness in the anatomical snuffbox should be x-rayed for possible fracture of the navicular. If the x-rays are negative, the wrist should be treated as if the athlete has suffered a sprain. If pain and disability persist for two to three weeks the wrist should be x-rayed again because a navicular fracture is notorious for not being readily visible on initial x-ray films. Navicular fractures frequently result in complications due to inadequate circulation. Therefore, all navicular fractures should be recognized and managed properly.

This same mechanism can cause a fracture to the distal end of the radius. This type of fracture will cause tenderness over the lower end of the radius and pain on hand movement. Complete fracture of the distal radius, in which the fragment is displaced upward or backward, is known as a **Colles' fracture.**

Wrist Support

The wrist is a frequent area to be supported by the use of athletic tape. The tape is used to restrict motion and support an injured or weakened wrist.

Figure 5-6 illustrates a common method of taping to restrict flexion of the wrist. Anchors are applied encircling the forearm and hand (#1 and #2). Strips #3 and #4 are applied from anchor to anchor in a crisscross ("X") manner. A series of three or four crisscrosses may be applied, depending upon the support needed (B).

The wrist taping procedure is locked by encircling strips of tape around the forearm and hand (C). If restriction of wrist extension is desired, then this same taping procedure is applied to the palm side of the hand and forearm. Occasionally, both sides of the wrist are supported at the same time.

INJURIES TO THE HAND

There are few sports in which the hands are not used in some manner. An athlete's hands are constantly exposed to various types of forced movements and direct trauma. As a result, a wide variety of athletic injuries to the hands can occur. Many are relatively minor and

Taping the Wrist

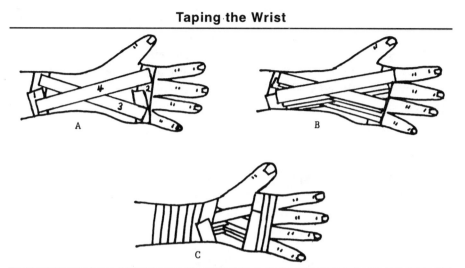

Fig. 5-6

are never reported to the coach or athletic trainer. Because there is a tendency by many athletes to underestimate or minimize injuries to this area of the body, injuries to the hands can develop into long-term impairment and permanent disability if not recognized and cared for properly. Therefore, it is important for you to be aware of signs and symptoms associated with the various injuries to the hand to avoid possible complications.

Contusions and Abrasions

These types of injuries are normally of little consequence; however, whenever the skin is broken about the hand, infection becomes a concern. All abrasions must be thoroughly cleaned and properly cared for in an attempt to prevent contamination and subsequent infection Contusion injuries resulting in hematoma formation about the hand are uncommon. The firmly fixed skin on the palmar surface allows little room for the pooling of blood. The loose mobile skin on the dorsum (back) of the hand, however, permits very marked swelling which normally does not last long.

Subungual hematoma. Direct trauma to the tips of the fingers or fingernails can cause blood to accumulate under the nail, which is called subungual hematoma. As the blood pools under the fingernail, a painful, throbbing, pressure develops which is usually relieved by drilling a hole in the nail and releasing the blood. Everyone has a favorite method of drilling a hole in the fingernail to relieve a subungual hematoma. Common methods involve the use of a nail drill, drilling with a sharp-pointed scalpel blade, or applying a red-hot paper clip to the nail.

Strains

Injuries involving the vast complex of tendons in the hand are not uncommon in athletics and are often missed on examination. The most common cause of these strains is overstretching or forcing the musculotendinous unit beyond its normal range of motion. The long flexor and extensor tendons are those most often strained. Symptomatically, these tendinous strains will present tenderness at the site of injury and increased pain on active and resistive contraction or passive stretching of the musculotendinous unit.

Baseball finger. Occasionally there will be a tendon rupture or avulsion of the tendinous attachment to the bone. This occurs most often at the distal phalanx, as the tendinous slip becomes narrow at the point of attachment. The extensor tendon may be injured by a blow to the tip of finger, forcing the distal interphalangeal joint into flexion and rupturing or partially rupturing the extensor tendon slip at the point of its insertion into the base of the terminal phalanx. This injury, commonly called a "baseball finger" or "mallet finger," is characterized by the athlete being unable to extend the distal phalanx. It is important that this injury be recognized and properly managed to prevent a permanent flexion deformity.

Profundus tendon rupture. Rupture or avulsion of the flexor digitorum profundus tendon from its attachment to the distal phalanx, is caused by a sudden extension of the DIP joint while held in flexion. This injury often occurs when an athlete gets the tip of a finger caught in a jersey or equipment as he or she attempts to grab another player. Therefore, this injury is often called a "jersey finger." On examination the athlete will be unable to actively flex the DIP joint. These athletes should be referred to medical attention to avoid any permanent functional deficit.

Sprains

Injuries involving the ligaments or ligamentous capsules surrounding the various joints of the hand are very common in athletic activity. This is especially true of the interphalangeal (IP) joints of the fingers. Sprains are normally the result of forced motion at a joint that stresses the supporting ligaments, causing varying degrees of damage. This forced motion is usually lateral motion, which stresses the collateral ligaments, or hyperextension, which stresses the anterior capsule. If this displacing force is strong enough or continuous, the joint will sublux or dislocate.

Symptomatically, sprains about the hand or digits will present tenderness at the site of injury and an increase in pain on reproduction of the stress that caused the injury. In addition, there are normally varying amounts of swelling, stiffness, and soreness surrounding the articulation that may take months to resolve. Depending on the amount of ligamentous damage, there may be varying amounts of instability associated with sprain injuries. If instability is recognized, the athlete should be referred to medical assistance.

The most common sprain of the hand is to the proximal interphalangeal (PIP) joints. When a finger is pulled or forced to the side, the supporting collateral ligaments or volar plate may be injured. This type of injury will exhibit tenderness over the collateral ligament involved, rapid swelling, and pain on passive stressing. Instability will be present on severe sprains. Inadequate evaluation and treatment of these injuries may lead to prolonged swelling, stiffness, pain, and loss of motion.

Skier's thumb. A sprain of the ulnar collateral ligament of the metacarpophalangeal (MCP) joint of the thumb is known as a "skier's thumb" or "gamekeeper's thumb." This commonly sprained ligament provides the stability necessary for normal grip and pinch. This type of injury is often overlooked or dismissed as a sprained thumb. If the ulnar collateral ligament is torn and inadequately cared for, continued instability, weakness of pinch, and recurrent effusion will probably occur. Characteristically this injury exhibits local tenderness over the ligament, joint effusion, and increased pain and instability on attempted abduction of the thumb.

Dislocations

The same mechanisms causing sprains may result in dislocations of the many joints of the hand. Dislocations involving the fingers occur more commonly than those in any other area of the body. These dislocations may remain displaced or may reduce spontaneously and appear as sprains on assessment. Finger dislocations are often readily reduced by the player, coach, or athletic trainer. It is a good practice to refer all athletes with dislocations, no matter how minor the injury may seem, to medical assistance. X-ray studies may be necessary to evaluate the presence of gross instability, ligament avulsion, or articular fracture. All too often athletes suffering dislocated fingers are treated casually and never seen by a physician. Inadequate treatment can lead to permanent instability and deformity of the joint.

Complete dislocations of the metacarpophalangeal joint of the thumb presents another problem in that the flexor tendons may loop around the metacarpal head, making closed reduction impossible. Dislocation of the thumb most often results from a fall that produces forceful hyperextension of the thumb on an extended hand. The usual deformity permits the phalanx to pass backward and rest upon the dorsal aspect of the thumb metacarpal. Dislocated thumbs should be reduced by a physician.

Fractures

Fractures of the hand frequently occur in athletics and result from the mechanisms of injury previously described. Because these fracture small bones, they are sometimes felt to be minor injuries and thus treated casually. However, finger stiffness, malunion, and functional disability may be disturbing consequences of hand fractures. Fractures of the metacarpals, which are more common than phalangeal fractures, usually result from a direct blow to the area or to the metacarpal head, which transmits the force down the shaft of the bone.

Fractures of the proximal and middle phalanges can result from a direct blow or the same mechanisms that cause dislocations, that is, forced lateral motion or hyperextension. A fracture of the shaft of a proximal phalanx, which is more commonly fractured than the other two phalanges, may result in V-shaped deformity or angulation. A fracture at the base of a proximal phalanx may be a combination fracture-dislocation. The distal phalanx is fractured most often by a crushing-type of mechanism.

Because of the subcutaneous nature of the long bones of the hand, you should be able to recognize the signs and symptoms which may indicate a fracture. Remember, it is a good practice to approach significant hand injuries as if there is a fracture until proven otherwise. Symptomatically, fractures will present tenderness at the site of injury, with pain elicited at the fracture site during longitudinal or transverse stress. In addition, deformity, crepitation, and a false joint may be present. All suspected fractures should be examined by a physician.

Hand Support

The thumb and/or fingers are frequently taped to provide support to an injured or weakened joint. Once again the objective is to restrict painful motion and provide support for the area.

Thumb Taping

Figure 5-7 illustrates the basic figure eight taping for support of the thumb. Use 1/2" - 1" tape to form a figure eight around the thumb and wrist (A). Start this taping procedure by laying the strip of tape at approximately the MCP joint (area marked by arrow) and allowing the tape to follow the natural contour of the area. Continuous figure eights are applied, moving up or down the thumb depending upon the injury, until support of the area is sufficient (B).

Caution: It is very easy to get this taping procedure too tight. The tape should be pulled off the roll as you come around the wrist and lightly placed around the thumb to avoid constriction.

Taping the Thumb (figure eight)

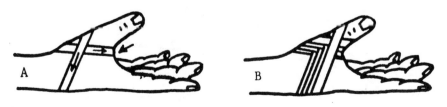

A

B

Fig. 5-7

Figure 5-8 illustrates a method of applying additional support to the base of the thumb. An anchor is placed around the hand (#1). Strips of tape are then applied from anchor to anchor encircling the base of the thumb and locked in place by lock strips around the hand (B). This tape job is often used in conjunction with the figure eight taping method.

Taping the Thumb (support at base)

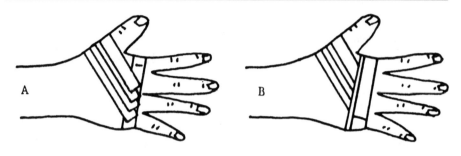

Fig. 5-8

Figure 5-9 illustrates a "checkrein" between the thumb and index finger. Narrow width tape is applied around the thumb and finger and then pinched together with a small piece of tape to form the checkrein. This procedure would be used to further prevent the thumb from abducting or going out away from the hand.

Checkrein for Thumb

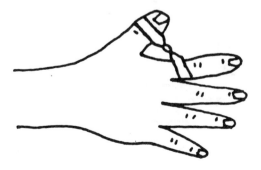

Fig. 5-9

Finger Taping

The metacarpophalangeal (MCP) joint is supported as illustrated in Figure 5-10. Using narrow tape, place an anchor around the hand (#1). Tape is then applied around the MCP joint, beginning and ending on the anchor strip (A). Continue applying strips until support is sufficient and lock in place with strips encircling the hand (B). Note the tape procedure illustrated is to restrict flexion of the MCP joint. If extension is the motion you want to limit, the taping procedure is applied to the palm side of the hand.

Taping MCP Joint

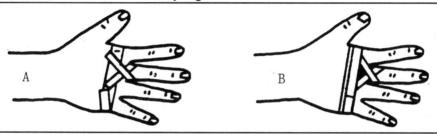

Fig. 5-10

The interphalangeal joints are normally supported by taping the injured finger to an uninjured one (Figure 5-11). By applying tape between the joints, the athlete still can flex and extend the fingers. If tape is placed over the joint, motion is further restricted. Figure 5-12 illustrates a method of applying a checkrein between two fingers. This method would be used if the athlete preferred to have the fingers taped apart.

Taping Fingers Together

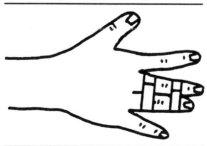

Fig. 5-11

Checkrein for Fingers

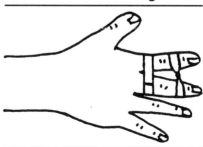

Fig. 5-12

HEAT RELATED CONDITIONS

Life-threatening situations in athletics are rare; however, they occasionally occur as the result of heat stress. The devastating effects of heat illness are needless and preventable. Anyone involved with athletes should have a basic understanding of the body's response to thermal exposure and how to prevent, recognize, and care for athletes suffering from heat stress conditions. Therefore, the final section of this manual will briefly discuss heat related conditions.

PHYSIOLOGICAL BASIS OF HEAT EXPOSURE

The human body is continually attempting to maintain a constant internal (core) temperature of 98° F (37° C). To maintain this constant temperature, heat lost must equal heat gain. If heat gain exceeds heat loss, the core temperature will rise; conversely, core temperature falls when heat loss exceeds heat production. The body has various mechanisms to gain as well as lose heat (Figure 6-1), and it is extremely important to maintain a balance between these mechanisms during athletic activity.

HEAT PRODUCTION

The body produces heat and energy during exercise and muscular exertion accompanying athletic activity. The greater the energy expenditure, the greater the heat production. A small amount of this heat is lost through vaporization of water in the air expired during respiration. However, most of the heat is carried by the blood into the circulatory system.

Mechanisms of Heat Gain and Loss

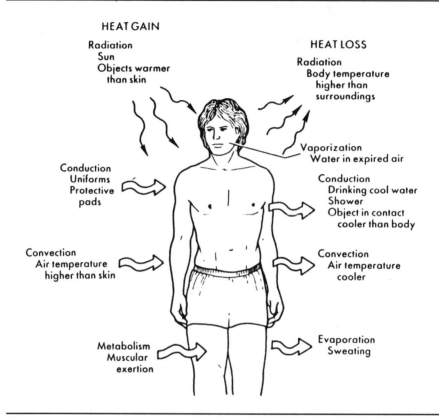

Fig. 6-1

HEAT GAIN

Heat can be gained by the body from the environment through **radiation, conduction,** and **convection.** We gain heat by radiation from the sun and surrounding objects that are warmer than the skins temperature. If the temperature of the air surrounding the athlete is higher than the athlete's temperature, he or she may gain heat through convection. An increase in core temperature may also occur through conduction or contact with protective equipment and uniforms.

HEAT DISSIPATION AND LOSS

As excess heat is produced or gained by the body, it must be eliminated or dissipated in order to keep the body temperature from reaching detrimental extremes. The body eliminates heat primarily by cutaneous vasodilation and sweating. When the core temperature rises, the body responds by increasing the peripheral blood flow in an attempt to transfer the heat from the core to the periphery. This brings an increase of body heat to the skin's surface, where it can be dissipated to the outside environment through radiation, convection, or conduction. This mechanism functions well as long as heat levels are not excessively high and the outside temperature is lower than the skin's surface.

The major portion of heat loss during athletics is through evaporation of sweat from the surface of the body. This is the body's major defense mechanism against overheating and serious heat illness. Our bodies are cooled only if the sweat evaporates. The effectiveness of this **sweating** and evaporation mechanism is strongly influenced by the relative humidity or the moisture in the air. That is, the lower the humidity, the faster the evaporation rate. As the relative humidity rises, the rate of the evaporation diminishes. Therefore, the combination of high temperature and high humidity decreases the body's ability to cool down, and increases the possibilities of heat related conditions. The rate of sweating also depends on the intensity of the activity, the physical condition of the athlete, how acclimated the athlete is, and the amount and type of clothing and equipment worn.

TEMPERATURE REGULATION

The thermoregulatory system of the body is controlled by the temperature regulatory center in the brain. The role of this center is analogous to that of the thermostat in a house. As information comes in that heat is being gained, the center automatically relays information to appropriate thermal receptors, and the mechanisms of vasodilation and sweating are initiated.

It is possible for an athlete's rate of heat gain and storage to become excessive in a very short period of time. If this occurs, it may overwhelm the body's mechanisms of heat loss. Such a situation can quickly develop into a serious heat illness. In addition, as the external temperature approaches that of the skin's surface or actually becomes higher, the heat dissipated by cutaneous vasodilation diminishes and may eventually cease completely. Body heat must then be dissipated primarily by the evaporation of sweat. If peripheral vasodilation is quite marked, the effective volume of the vascular system is decreased, and the heart must increase its output to compensate and maintain adequate blood flow. This is accomplished by an increase in both heart rate and stroke volume. Unfortunately, at least some degree of vaso-motor control of the cutaneous vessels may be lost during heat stress. The result is pooling of blood in the extremities. As blood is progres-sively shunted into the periphery, less and less blood flows to the in-ternal organs and central nervous system.

Another important physiological consideration is the volume of sweat lost from the body. Profuse sweating can cause excessive losses of body water, which can result in a decreased blood volume and de-hydration and a decreased rate of sweating and cooling by evapora-tion. If this water is not replaced, circulatory collapse (shock) may re-sult from the continuing decrease in blood volume. As sweating de-creases there is also a decrease in evaporative cooling, which can cause an excessive rise in core temperature. As water loss becomes extremely excessive, the mechanism of sweating is shut off to maintain or con-serve blood volume. When this happens, internal body temperature soars, giving way to a serious heat condition, heatstroke.

HEAT RELATED CONDITIONS

Three specific heat illnesses or syndromes can result from ther-mal exposure; (1) **heat cramps**, (2) **heat exhaustion**, and (3) **heatstroke**. These three are listed in order from the least serious to the most seri-ous. Each is normally caused by the same set of circumstances; that is, strenuous activity in a combination of hot and humid weather, result-ing in a loss of body water and a derangement of the body's thermoregu-latory system. Although the cause of these heat-related conditions is normally the same, each represents a different bodily reaction to exces-sive heat, with their own set of signs and symptoms and treatment pro-cedures. It is extremely important to be familiar with signs and symp-toms that indicate the development of heat illnesses, as well as emer-gency measures necessary to adequately care for athletes suffering from serious heat stress.

It is important to remember that heat cramps and heat exhaustion can lead to heatstroke. This is especially true when working with athletes. In most types of activity, a person will voluntarily stop working and seek relief from the heat when either heat cramps or heat exhaustion appear to be developing. Athletes, on the other hand, especially highly competitive or motivated athletes, are more likely to continue working out or exercising even though symptoms may be developing. Athletes in a sport such as football are required to wear heavy protective equipment and uniforms that cover much of the body and add to the problem of heat dissipation. Athletes are also engaged in strenuous activity under the influence of the coaches' or trainers' philosophies concerning the number of breaks, availability of water, and the intensity of the exercise sessions. All of these factors are pertinent to the development of heat-related conditions.

Heat Cramps

Heat cramps are the least serious of the three heat illnesses. These cramps are painful spasms of skeletal muscles. Past training literature suggested that heat cramps are caused by salt or electrolyte loss. More recent literature, however, suggests that heat cramps result from a fluid volume problem and can normally be prevented by providing unlimited amounts of water to athletes throughout activity in hot weather.

When heat cramps do occur, they normally accompany strenuous physical activity and profuse sweating in hot weather. The most common muscles involved are the calf muscles or abdominals, but any of the voluntary muscles can be affected by a sudden and painful spasm or cramp. Heat cramps may be mild, with slight cramping, or they may be quite severe and incapacitating, with intense pain. Athletes suffering heat cramps are normally alert and oriented to their surroundings. The skin will be wet and warm as a result of excessive sweating. The body temperature, pulse, and respiratory rate should be normal or slightly elevated.

In most cases heat cramps are not a serious problem and can be relieved by slowly stretching the contracted muscle. The application of ice, firm pressure or gentle massage to the area may facilitate relief. The athlete should also be encouraged to drink liquids. Many times the athlete will resume activity after alleviation of the muscle spasms;

however, a severe episode of heat cramps may require the athlete to avoid further exertion for a longer period of time, perhaps 12 to 24 hours. Should heat cramps frequently recur in the same athlete, additional assessment of specific causes is warranted, and medical referral may be necessary. Remember, athletes who suffer heat cramps should be closely observed as this condition may precipitate heat exhaustion or heatstroke.

Heat Exhaustion

Heat exhaustion is probably the most common condition caused by exertion in hot weather. The physiological basis for heat exhaustion has been previously described; that is, peripheral vasodilation, loss of vasomotor control, and vascular pooling. Because of this peripheral vascular collapse, these athletes are suffering from an abnormally decreased volume of blood circulating in the body.

It is important to recognize the signs and symptoms associated with heat exhaustion and be able to differentiate them from those associated with heatstroke. Figure 6-2 illustrates the main signs and symptoms associated with both conditions.

Main Signs and Symptoms Associated with Heat Exhaustion and Heatstroke

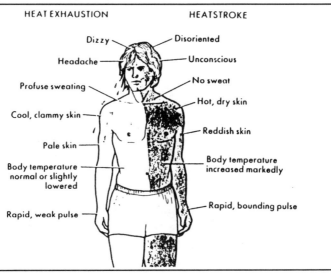

HEAT EXHAUSTION

HEATSTROKE

Dizzy

Headache

Profuse sweating

Cool, clammy skin

Pale skin

Body temperature normal or slightly lowered

Rapid, weak pulse

Disoriented

Unconscious

No sweat

Hot, dry skin

Reddish skin

Body temperature increased markedly

Rapid, bounding pulse

Fig. 6-2

Heat exhaustion is characterized by profuse sweating, which makes the skin wet, cool, and clammy. The skin may also appear pale or grey. The decrease in blood volume normally results in headache, weakness, dizziness, fatigue, nausea, and occasionally unconsciousness. The athlete may be disoriented, and heat cramps may accompany this condition. The body temperature is usually normal or slightly below normal, and the respiration usually fast and shallow. Heat exhaustion may lead to complete collapse of the thermoregulatory system if not properly identified and treated.

Heat exhaustion is normally not life threatening, but proper medical care is required. The athlete should be treated as if in shock; that is, taken out of the hot environment and placed supine with the feet elevated. Remove as much equipment and uniform as possible. The cooling process can be assisted by sponging or toweling the athlete with cool water. If the athlete is conscious, allow him or her to drink cool fluids. The athlete will normally feel better in a short period of time; however, should symptoms persist, the athlete should be transported to a medical facility. Athletes suffering heat exhaustion should be withdrawn from further activity for the remainder of that day and closely observed.

Heatstroke

Heatstroke (sunstroke) is the least common of the heat related conditions but certainly the most serious. Heatstroke occurs when the thermoregulatory system of the body is completely overwhelmed or the volume of circulating blood becomes so low that the sweating mechanism is shut off to conserve depleted fluid levels. When either of these occur, the body temperature rises rapidly to dangerous and ultimately fatal levels. The body temperature may go over 106° F (41.1° C).

Heatstroke is a severe medical emergency and must be recognized and treated immediately. This condition is characterized by hot, dry skin and a rising temperature. The athlete's skin is normally reddened or flushed. As the temperature rises, the pulse becomes very rapid and strong. Initially the athlete may experience headache, dizziness, and weakness, which are often followed by convulsions and unconsciousness.

The immediate emergency care for an athlete exhibiting signs of heatstroke is to reduce the body temperature as quickly as possible by any means available. This may include cooling the body by placing ice or cold towels around the body, immersing the athlete in cold water, directing a fan at the athlete, or sponging the body with cool water or alcohol. Remove clothing and equipment to prevent the retention of body heat. If the athlete is conscious, allow him or her to drink cool water. Athletes suffering from heatstroke are critically ill and must be taken to a medical facility as soon as possible. Aggressive efforts to lower the body temperature should continue during the referral and transfer process.

PREVENTIVE MEASURES

Following is a brief discussion of several important measures you can take to prevent or reduce the impact of heat stress on the body.

Heat acclimation. This is the process of becoming accustomed to athletic activity in hot weather. It improves the circulatory and sweating responses, and facilitates the dissipation of heat. Heat acclimation helps minimize changes in body temperature. Acclimation renders the athlete more capable of adapting to or tolerating the stresses of heat and is the most efficient method of handling increased external temperatures.

For heat acclimation to occur, athletes must workout or exercise in hot weather. It is best for an athlete to acclimate gradually over a period of time before scheduled practices or an athletic season begins. Each athlete will acclimate at a different rate. Further, the athlete in good condition is capable of more work in the heat and will acclimate more rapidly than the nonconditioned athlete. It is believed that optimal acclimation requires an athlete to exercise between one to two hours daily. With this type of a schedule, acclimation is usually well developed in five to seven and complete in 12 to 14 days. In addition, athletes should have adequate access to water during the acclimation period, because withholding fluids significantly retards this process.

Recording temperature and humidity. It is important to measure the temperature and humidity during hot weather activity. These measurements should be made before and during training sessions, and adjustments or modifications in activity made if so indicated. These adjustments include decreasing intensity levels of activity, providing more breaks and fluids, eliminating unnecessary clothing, or delaying or postponing practices until conditions improve.

There are several methods of monitoring the temperature and humidity. One of the easiest methods is to obtain these readings from the local weather bureau and chart them on a graph such as Figure 6-3. This type of guide was developed from weather data gathered at the time of heatstroke fatalities occurring in football. Any combination of environmental conditions in the white zone would be considered safe. Conditions in the lightly shaded zone would be a warning area, and the athletes would need to be carefully observed for signs and symptoms of heat illness. The darker shaded zone would be the danger area. If conditions in this zone were present, practices should be modified or

Weather Guide for the Prevention of Heat Conditions

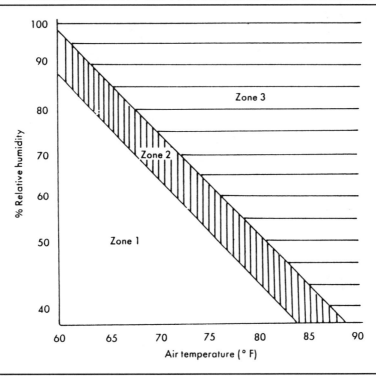

Fig. 6-3

postponed, and athletes closely observed. Note that humidity is a significant factor, even in the presence of moderate temperatures.

Fluid replacement. Water is one of the major necessities of life. As previously discussed, decreased body fluid associate with profuse sweating diminishes the available blood volume and sweating necessary for body cooling. Fluids must be provided. Athletes should have unlimited and easy access to water during all athletic activity in hot weather. It is better for athletes to drink small amounts frequently than to schedule a break every hour or so, when they may gulp large amounts of water. Deliberately withholding water from athletes for purposes of weight loss may be extremely hazardous in hot weather.

Medical history. Obtain a complete medical history, including any previous heat illnesses or problems caused by the heat. Has the athlete ever fainted from excessive heat? Has the athlete ever had any sweating problems? Athletes who have suffered previous heat related problems may have some permanent damage to the thermoregulatory center and are more prone to future heat disorders.

Physical condition. Evaluate the general physical condition of the athlete. Has he or she been working out in the heat? Inquire about the duration and intensity of work and training activities. Athletes in poor physical condition are candidates for heat illness. In addition, athletes who are overfat have an appreciable decreased ability to dissipate heat.

Clothing and uniforms. In hot or humid weather, clothing and uniforms should be light-weight, loose fitting, and light colored to reflect the sun. Porous or net shirts expose more of the body surface for evaporation of sweat and dissipation of body heat. Avoid the use of long stockings, long sleeves, excess clothing, and sweat suits during hot weather activity. This type of clothing can seriously limit heat loss by reducing evaporative cooling. Rubberized clothing should never be used in hot weather, as it does not allow the evaporation of sweat and dissipation of body heat.

Rest periods. Provide rest periods during hot weather activities to dissipate accumulated body heat. If possible, athletes should rest in cool, shaded areas with some air movement. Loosen or remove heavy or tight-fitting jerseys to expose more skin surface. Allow football players to remove their helmets. In areas where hot weather conditions are especially severe, unique arrangements for moving air, such as placement of large fans, may be required.

Weight charts. Weight charts can facilitate the detection of an athlete who may be more susceptible to heat stress. Daily measurements of weight loss, which mainly reflects water loss, should be taken and recorded. Athletes losing excessive amounts of weight each day, in excess of 3% of their body weight, which is not made up in a 24-hour period, should be observed carefully; they may be candidates for heat illness.

Diet. A well-balanced diet is essential to athletic activity and will normally replenish any electrolytes or body minerals lost during hot weather. For example, sufficient salt replacement will normally occur with a balanced diet. It is not recommended that athletes ingest salt tablets.

SUMMARY

The body's response to thermal exposure is basically one of maintaining heat balance; that is, the same amount of heat must be lost as produced or gained by the body during activity in hot weather, primarily by cutaneous vasodilation and sweating. Peripheral blood flow is increased to transfer heat from the core of the body to the periphery, where it can be dissipated. The evaporation of sweat from the skin's surface is the body's major defense mechanism against overheating. There are many factors, both internal and external, that influence or affect these two important heat dissipating mechanisms. Whenever abnormal demands are placed on the thermoregulatory system and the heat gained exceeds that lost, athletes are subjected to the effects of heat-related conditions. These conditions can be significantly reduced through heat acclimation, adequate water replacement, and the awareness of various factors imposed on the athlete by the combinations of exercise, environment, and clothing.

Heat-related conditions include heat cramps, heat exhaustion, and heatstroke. Heat cramps are the least serious, heat exhaustion the most common, and heatstroke the most serious. Each of these is caused by basically the same set of circumstances, but each represents a different bodily reaction to excessive heat. It is extremely important to be familiar with signs and symptoms that indicate the development of these heat conditions, as well as emergency measures that should be immediately initiated should they occur.